LIVING IN THE
MIRACULOUS

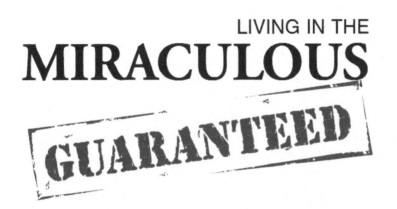

Jim Hockaday

Living In The Miraculous
© 2003 by Jim Hockaday
P. O. Box 729
Castle Rock, CO 80104

All rights reserved. No part of this book may be reproduced, stored in a retrieval system, or transmitted in any form or by any means without expressed written permis-sion of the author.

All Scripture quotations unless otherwise noted are from the New King James Version. Copyright©1979, 1980, 1982 by Thomas Nelson, Inc. Used by permission. All rights reserved.

Other Scripture Quotations:
New American Standard Bible (NAS) ©1960, 1977 The Lockman Foundation

Holy Bible: New International Version ©1973, 1978, 1984 by the International Bible Society. Used by Permission of Zondervan Publishing House. All rights reserved.

The Miracle of The Scarlet Thread
All rights reserved
Copyright ©1981 by Sounds of the Trumpet, Inc. Destiny Group Publishing
P.O. Box 310
Shippensburg, PA 17257

Published by Jim Hockaday Ministries, Inc.
ISBN: 978-1-7343472-0-3

Original Cover Art: Tina Winford
Interior Design: Cathleen Kwas
Editor: Dr. Larry Keefauver

TABLE OF CONTENTS

Foreword—Why Not?...v
Introduction—Live in the Miraculous!........................7
Chapter 1—Think Right..13
Chapter 2—Expectation Births Miracles...................31
Chapter 3—In the Beginning, God!..............................45
Chapter 4—Faith Acts on God's Covenant
  Promises 61
Chapter 5—Jehovah's Names Guarantee the
  Miraculous!..89
Chapter 6—God's Miraculous Ways 115
Chapter 7—Practicing the Reality of the
  Miraculous 141
Chapter 8—Abiding in the Vine................................161
Conclusion—The Miraculous—Guaranteed!...........191

Foreword

WHY NOT?

You are in for a spiritual treat! Your inner man will leap for joy as you read and then act in faith on God's Word as it's uncovered in Jim Hockaday's wonderful and easy to understand explanation of how to live in the miraculous.

You can have the mindset of Jesus.

You can see the same signs and wonders witnessed by the early church in your daily walk with Jesus.

You can experience the power of the Holy Spirit working in and through you to do what the Father wills in your life.

Why not experience the miraculous *now*? Guaranteed!

When will the miraculous happen for you? The surprising truth is this: *you don't have to wait!* You don't have to wait until you understand all the deeper truths of Scripture. You don't have to wait until you reach a certain esoteric level of spiritual knowledge. You don't have to wait until there's less sin and more holiness in your life. You don't have to try harder in your prayer life.

You don't have to wait until Jesus comes!

In fact, your effort will never produce the miraculous! So, when will you live in it?

- When you start reading this exciting book by Jim Hockaday.
- When you start trusting God's Word for your life.
- When you really believe that what God promised is for you instead of just for others!

I want to challenge you to read *Living In The Miraculous* immediately. Don't let another day pass before you step out of the natural and into the supernatural. Don't wait another minute for the ordinary to become extraordinary—begin to exercise your faith *now!*

Jim's clear, insightful, biblical teaching has deepened my faith and increased my walk in the miraculous. Now it's your turn! Enjoy!

Dr. Larry Keefauver
May 16, 2003
Orlando, Florida

Introduction

LIVE IN THE MIRACULOUS!

THROUGH WRONG CONCEPTS of God and legalistic religious ideas, most of us have forfeited many opportunities to live in the supernatural. It is safe to say that nothing is ever accomplished where there is no action. Working with and responding to God is learned through a revelation of God's loving desire for man.

Throughout the Word of God, truth is revealed which assures us of God's ever-present help. Imagine learning and understanding God's heart for the miraculous so well that our bold confident actions of faith would manifest God's love to the world. Is it true that all things with God are really possible?

We'll never know until we dare to believe and act.

In every generation a time and a requirement arises for greatness. One person or more, who will dare to brave the unthinkable, defies the odds by going beyond the status quo. Throughout the Old Testament, we see glimpses of God's investment into this world. Many brave-hearted men and women responded to God's ability to effect change in the earth.

These faithful men and women exhibited a spirit of daringness and confidence. Daniel revealed this same spirit, "But the people who know their God shall be strong, and carry out great exploits" (Dan. 11:32). What quality separated these men and women from all the rest of humanity? Simply this: they trusted and confided in God in ways different from today. What did they know *then* that we don't *now*?

The Jesus Factor

Two thousand years ago there was a man born in Bethlehem, raised in Nazareth in the region of Judea who understood His requirement for greatness. His name was Jesus, who was and is the Christ, the Son of the Living God. This world has forever been branded with His standard. He is the reason we were created.

In His time, Jesus stood alone as the Son of God revealed. Not since the days of Adam and Eve, before sin entered the world, has this planet and its occupants known the true purpose and meaning of life. Jesus was the divine expression of creation's original purpose. His dominion, love, authority and sinlessness gave all of creation the hope of complete redemption. "For the creation was subjected to futility, not willingly, but because of Him who subjected it in hope; because the creation itself also will be delivered from the bondage of corruption into the glorious liberty of the children of God" (Rom. 8:20-21).

In my second book, *Until I Come*, I explored the mind of Christ. I proposed that since we are the body of Christ—the head of the church, it would be expedient for us to know what the head is thinking. Our success in being His body is directly linked to understanding our responsibilities in Christ and God's ability to empower us to fulfill them.

What a wonderful revelation it is to know who you are in Christ, your divine authority in the earth and God's great love solution for you and the world. Without that revelation, you will never envision God working in and through you to produce change in you and others.

Yet, we must ask ourselves...

- How do we respond to difficulties?
- When we take our place in Christ, do we hope that God will come through for us?

- Is our boldness or a lack of it a reflection of our trust in God?
- As co-laborers in Christ, are we seeing the miraculous in our lives and in the church?
- Can we really know the mind of God?
- What is God's perspective of reality and how can we live in that reality?
- Is He seeing things different than we do?
- Are we confident enough to trust Him with our lives?
- Are we really sure that He will come through for us?

It's Time for Great Exploits!

In Daniel 11:32, these amazing words challenge us, "Those who do wickedly against the covenant he shall corrupt with flattery; but **the people who know their God shall be strong, and carry out great exploits**." If knowing God is proportionate to showing strength and doing exploits, can we distinguish between knowing about and actually knowing Him? We must never separate our faith in God from our fellowship with God.

We read in Judges 2:8-10, "Joshua son of Nun, the servant of the LORD, died at the age of a hundred and ten. And they buried him in the land of his inheritance, at Timnath Heres in the hill country of Ephraim, north of Mount Gaash. After that whole generation had been gathered to their fathers, another generation grew up, who knew neither the LORD nor what he had done for Israel" (NIV). That generation had lost both the knowledge of God and intimacy with Him.

Let's determine to be a generation who knows God intimately and understands what to expect from Him. If we are unsure of what God can do and don't know Him well enough to trust Him, then we will always be lacking His ability. Let us never be timid about who we are in Christ. Isn't it time for a remnant of the body of Christ to rise above the dangers and fears of these last days? May we always enter life's battles knowing with certainty "that the battle is the Lord's."

In this book you will...

- Discover God's mindset
- Learn how to expect the incredible and the miraculous
- Uncover the authority for the miraculous that God has deposited in you
- Understand the power released in God's names
- See God's way of doing things
- Begin to practice God's reality for your life
- Be released from the bondage of works to the freedom of abiding in *the* Vine
- Get ready! You are about to step into the incredible, see the invisible, and...
- Do the miraculous with God through Christ Jesus!

Chapter 1

THINK RIGHT

ONE OF THE CRAZES IN THE MOVIE industry today seems to be the exploitation of reality shows—real people doing really crazy things for money. I like the concept of reality shows that endeavor to create real environments without any special effects. The movie industry for decades has produced thrilling shows with stunts that are only real to the imagination. I believe it's time for the church to produce its own reality shows.

Is Your God Too Small?

As the church, we should be revealing to the world the true, awesome nature of God. Maybe it's time we had reality checks on our concept of God. A bestselling classic by J.B. Phillips, *Your God is Too Small*, describes the mindset of most Christians. If it's true that what we think about, believe and act on will produce and shape our tomorrows, then are we willing to investigate what it is that we really embrace and believe?

The Apostle Paul challenges us in Ephesians 3:20-21, "Now to Him who is able to do exceedingly abundantly above all that we ask or think, according to the power that works in us, to Him be glory in the church by Christ Jesus to all generations, forever and ever. Amen." I believe in this verse God challenges the New Testament church in much the same way He challenged Israel with Malachi 3:10. God challenged the children of Israel to prove Him concerning financial blessings. Malachi 3:10 declares, "Bring ye all the tithes into the storehouse, that there may be meat in mine house, and prove me now herewith, saith the LORD of hosts, if I will not open you the windows of heaven, and pour you out a blessing, that there shall not be room enough to receive it" (KJV).

This is an awesome passage when you consider that you cannot out give God. If someone were to take God seriously, they would faithfully give their tithe and generously give offerings with complete confidence that their return would be supernatural.

So, in Ephesians 3:20-21, God issues a challenge to us in the supernatural realm much like He challenges us in the financial realm through Malachi. Paul begins by affirming, "Now unto Him who is able *to do*."

God Is Able *To Do...*

Aren't you glad that God is able *to do*? Jesus revealed that the things which are impossible with men are possible with God. Having knowledge of how someone is able to help you is very important to your response. Notice the four words that Paul uses to describe how God is able to do.

1. **Exceedingly** means, exceptional in amount, quality, or degree.
2. **Abundantly** means, an ample or overflowing quantity.
3. **Above** means, exceeding in number, quantity, or size.
4. And **All** simply means all. **All** refers to anything felt, thought or imagination within us. What God does goes far beyond anything we can reason in our finite minds or thoughts. **All** shatters every barrier and overflows every bank. **All** breaks through any hindrance, stronghold or boundary that has been set by us or the world.

Now you can see how serious God is about performing His word. Here comes the challenge. God's awesome display of His ability in your life is in reference to how big you can ask or think. One day as I was meditating on this verse, I said to the Lord, "I trust you were serious about this verse, because I can think pretty big."

God is endeavoring to show us how far out of our box He is willing to go to satisfy our faith. The Amplified Bible says, "Infinitely beyond our highest prayers, thoughts, desires, hopes or dreams...." Let's face it, at times we put God in a box of our own experience and finite expectations. Remember this:

We can't ask too big or out think God. The power that is at work in us qualifies us to actually see the results of our faith.

Don't Be Deceived!

After thinking about this scripture and contemplating the possibilities, is it any wonder why the devil works so hard to infiltrate the mind of the believer with religion, doubt and unbelief. Can you imagine the impact a society would feel if Christians around the world dared to believe this verse?

Now that I have both your attention and curiosity, let's look at the context for verses 20 and 21. Take time to read this slowly and out loud. Let the Word penetrate both your mind and spirit.

> *To me, who am less than the least of all the saints, this grace was given, that I should preach among the Gentiles the unsearchable riches of Christ, and to make all see what is*

the fellowship of the mystery, which from the beginning of the ages has been hidden in God who created all things through Jesus Christ; to the intent that now the manifold wisdom of God might be made known by the church to the principalities and powers in the heavenly places, according to the eternal purpose which He accomplished in Christ Jesus our Lord, in whom we have boldness and access with confidence through faith in Him. Therefore I ask that you do not lose heart at my tribulations for you, which is your glory.

For this reason I bow my knees to the Father of our Lord Jesus Christ, from whom the whole family in heaven and earth is named, that He would grant you, according to the riches of His glory, to be strengthened with might through His Spirit in the inner man, that Christ may dwell in your hearts through faith; that you, being rooted and grounded in love, may be able to comprehend with all the saints what is the width and length and depth and height— to know the love of Christ which passes knowledge; that you may be filled with all the fullness of God. (Eph. 3:8-19)

Paul recognized the importance of making known the manifold wisdom of God. The great mystery of the church had been revealed. It was time for the church to come to the understanding of what she possessed. Do you see how important knowledge is to the believer?

In the first chapter of Ephesians Paul prayed that the Father of our Lord Jesus Christ would grant the church wisdom and revelation in the knowledge of God. Paul continues by praying that the eyes of our understanding would be enlightened. Remember, if there were no adversary and the world wasn't so adversely contrary to the ways of God, there wouldn't be so much opposition to our thinking as Paul makes mention of in 2 Corinthians 4:3-4, "But even if our gospel is veiled, it is veiled to those who are perishing, whose minds the god of this age has blinded, who do not believe, lest the light of the gospel of the glory of Christ, who is the image of God, should shine on them."

If the devil aims his deception at the unbeliever to keep him from becoming saved, then why wouldn't he also attempt to blind our minds to the wonders of our salvation?

The devil has never changed his tactics. The first encounter man experienced with the devil was in the Garden of Eden. His plan of attack is the exact same today. The reason for this book is to help you understand and then overcome the enemy's attack.

> *Now the serpent was more crafty than any of the wild animals the LORD God had made.*
>
> *He said to the woman, "Did God really say, 'You must not eat from any tree in the garden'?"*

> *The woman said to the serpent, "We may eat fruit from the trees in the garden, but God did say, 'You must not eat fruit from the tree that is in the middle of the garden, and you must not touch it, or you will die!"*
>
> *"You will not surely die," the serpent said to the woman* (Gen. 3:1-4 NIV).

First, the devil questioned what God said. The number one reason for his deception is to keep you ignorant of God's will and plan for your life.

Second, the serpent questioned whether or not God would do what he said. This scenario just described the contents for active faith. When you know what God has said, and you are confident that God will do what He said, you are ready for action. It's so important for you to possess the mind of God!

When Paul prayed that the eyes of our understanding would be opened, he prayed this so that we would know the hope of our calling, the glorious riches of our inheritance and what is the greatness of His mighty power that is toward us, which He worked in Christ when He raised Him from the dead and seated Him in heavenly places.

In the past thirty years, the body of Christ has had some of the greatest teaching filled with revelation that the church has ever had. Such tremendous knowledge has been made available. Yet with all this teaching there has not been a balance of the demonstration of the word taught.

We know a lot about God, yet few really know Him. What makes an earthly father-son relationship so wonderful is that the time of fellowship between the two of them builds absolute trust with each other. It's this security in trust or faith that means so much to a person's stability. Yet, we see great instability within the church. We must ask...

- Why does the church run so quickly to the world for its solutions?
- Do we really doubt that God will help us?

From our verses in Genesis you can understand that the devil will work hard to keep you from knowing the truth—God's plan, will and blessings for your life. If he can't keep you ignorant, then he will work hard to make you insecure about God's faithfulness to do what He said He would do. You can quote all day long that you believe God is faithful, although, when push comes to shove and you're in the heat of battle, how do you act?

Are You Thinking Big or Limiting God?

There is a great Old Testament story that illustrates whether or not we are thinking big enough or limiting God.

> *The company of the prophets said to Elisha, "Look, the place where we meet with you is*

too small for us. Let us go to the Jordan, where each of us can get a pole; and let us build a place there for us to live."

And he said, "Go."

Then one of them said, "Won't you please come with your servants?"

"I will," Elisha replied. And he went with them.

They went to the Jordan and began to cut down trees. As one of them was cutting down a tree, the iron axhead fell into the water. "Oh, my lord," he cried out, "it was borrowed!"

The man of God asked, "Where did it fall?" When he showed him the place, Elisha cut a stick and threw it there, and made the iron float.

"Lift it out," he said. Then the man reached out his hand and took it. (2 Kings 6:1-7 NIV).

Be honest with yourself. Ask yourself...

- Would you have cut a twig from a tree and by throwing it into the water where the ax head fell, raised it up?
- What would have been your response?
- Would you have asked everyone to pitch in so you would have enough money to buy a new one?
- Or, would you at least go to the home of the one who you borrowed the ax from

and ask for some time to pay for the lost ax?

In one sense you could say that there is nothing wrong with any of these solutions except one thing: *they are all based on what you can do.*

How often do we bring God into the equation? Most of us exhaust every possibility that we or others can think of before going to God as a last resort. Paul said in Rom 8:5-8,

"For those who live according to the flesh set their minds on the things of the flesh, but those who live according to the Spirit, the things of the Spirit. For to be carnally minded is death, but to be spiritually minded is life and peace. Because the carnal mind is enmity against God; for it is not subject to the law of God, nor indeed can be."

Paul reminds us about how our own affections restrict us, "You are not restricted by us, but you are restricted by your own affections" (2 Cor. 6:12). When the natural things of life outweigh the things of God you are prone to act naturally. You don't have to have your head in the clouds all the time to be spiritual. However, there must be an awareness of God in your soul. Very simply, God-awareness comes when your thoughts are centered around and on God.

Isn't it interesting that Elisha didn't have a word from the Lord instructing him to do what he did? It's amazing to see this Old Testament man of God conceptualizing the possibilities of the supernatural. He made it look so easy, didn't he? Has God's plan of redemption destined us to struggle through life, never knowing how we're going to make it?

Are you ready for a challenge? Let's look in Genesis 3 and 4 to finish our discussion on these thoughts. Gen 3:7-13 reads:

> *Then the eyes of both of them were opened, and they knew that they were naked; and they sewed fig leaves together and made themselves coverings. And they heard the sound of the LORD God walking in the garden in the cool of the day, and Adam and his wife hid themselves from the presence of the LORD God among the trees of the garden.*
>
> *Then the LORD God called to Adam and said to him, "Where are you?" So he said, "I heard Your voice in the garden, and I was afraid because I was naked; and I hid myself." And He said, "Who told you that you were naked? Have you eaten from the tree of which I commanded you that you should not eat?" Then the man said, "The woman whom You gave to be with me, she gave me of the tree, and I ate." And the LORD God said to the woman, "What is this you have done?" The woman said, "The serpent deceived me, and I ate."*

I trust you understand that by the seventh verse Adam and Eve had already sinned by disobeying God. This would make them sinners by nature. God had warned them in the second chapter and the seventeenth verse that, in the day that they partake of the forbidden fruit, they would die. The margin in my Bible says, "in dying thou shalt die," signifying that there would be a double death.

Now we know that they didn't die physically immediately, but they did die spiritually. Spiritual death is simply separation from God. They inherited the nature of the devil. They became like him, sinful by nature. This is the reason why a man or woman born in sin needs more than just forgiveness. They need a change in nature.

What every person needs is to be born again, to be changed into the very nature of Jesus Christ, i.e. to be fully restored to "the image of God." I want to make sure you understand that when they sinned, Adam and Eve were separated from God in their spirit. Genesis 3:8 is shocking. The Bible records that Adam and Eve heard the sound of God walking in the cool of the day. I thought they were spiritually dead, how then can they hear God? The next part of verse eight is also amazing. They hid themselves from the presence of the Lord. Is it possible that these "fallen, sinful" beings recognized the presence of God?

Sensing God's Presence

I had a very interesting experience while traveling with the Rhema Singers and Band as we accompanied Rev. Kenneth Hagin in his meetings. We were singing and helping Brother Hagin at camp meeting in the late 80's. In addition to singing in the group, I would stay close to Brother Hagin if he needed any help while ministering to the people. The camp meeting stage was very long and the stairs were at the back of the stage. Brother Hagin decided to go down to the main floor where the people were.

Usually I followed directly behind him. This night Cindy, one of the members of the group who helped with the modesty cloths got right in behind Brother Hagin as we were walking down, so I was behind her. As the three of us walked toward the stairs, I began to smell a beautiful fragrance. Of course, I assumed it was coming from Cindy. As we reached the main floor and began walking toward the people, the fragrance became much stronger.

I began to think to myself, "Wow, Cindy, you really put the perfume on tonight. Maybe she had a date afterwards." Now we were out in front of the people, and Brother Hagin said, "Does anyone smell that?"

I thought, "Hey, Brother Hagin smells Cindy too!" Then Brother Hagin said, "That fragrance is the fragrance of God."

All the time I thought I was smelling Cindy. I was so thrilled that I was having an experience with God that I forgot about my duties and sat down and enjoyed that fragrance. How many Christians go through life without ever experiencing the presence of God?

The Glory of God will come into a meeting and most of us will be thinking, "If anything is here, I don't know it." Do you see the significance of Adam and Eve recognizing the presence of God, and they are sinners? If this doesn't challenge us enough, look at verse nine and the following. God says to Adam, "Where are you?"

Adam not only hears, but also responds to God beginning a dialogue with complete sentences. Let me remind you that Adam is a sinner. Not just a little sinner, half a sinner, or just a beginner sinner. Adam is spiritually separated from God. How then can he hear from God like this?

Before answering this question go to Genesis 4.

> *Now Adam knew Eve his wife, and she conceived and bore Cain, and said, "I have acquired a man from the LORD." Then she bore again, this time his brother Abel. Now Abel was a keeper of sheep, but Cain was a tiller of the ground. And in the process of time it came to pass that Cain brought an offering of the fruit of the ground to the LORD. Abel also brought of the firstborn of his flock and of their fat. And the LORD respected Abel and his offering, but He did not respect Cain and his offering. And Cain was very angry, and his countenance fell.*
>
> *So the LORD said to Cain, "Why are you angry? And why has your countenance fallen? If you do well, will you not be accepted? And if you do not do well, sin lies at the door. And its desire is for you, but you*

> *should rule over it."* Now Cain talked with Abel his brother; and it came to pass, when they were in the field, that Cain rose up against Abel his brother and killed him.
>
> Then the LORD said to Cain, "Where is Abel your brother?" He said, "I do not know. Am I my brother's keeper?" And He said, "What have you done? The voice of your brother's blood cries out to Me from the ground. (Gen. 4:1-11)

Correct me if I'm wrong, but here we have second-generation sinners. Cain and Abel must be in their teens to be responsible enough to handle the jobs they were given by Adam and Eve. So we could safely say that fifteen or so years have passed since Adam's disobedience in the Garden of Eden.

What's amazing is that Cain who is contemplating murder is hearing the voice of God like Adam and Eve in Genesis 3. As born again, spirit-filled believers we pray for hours and get excited if we hear one word, yet we don't know what it means. We've been made righteous, restored to favor with God and we're seated at the right hand of God in Christ, you'd think that if any one could hear from God it would be us, God's children. What's the missing link?

When you consider Adam and Eve and their sons, you can immediately see that sin had not yet become proficient. They were experiencing all kinds of interesting battles that they had not known before. Their minds were still tuned in enough to what they had known of God and what was right, yet this new sin nature began to lead them into all kinds of new emotions and desires. This sounds like what Paul described in Galatians 5:17, "the flesh lusts against the spirit, and the spirit against the flesh, and these are contrary to one another."

We Need an Awareness of God!

Adam and Eve retained enough of the mind of God that they were able to hear God clearly. God is a spirit and so is every human being. Adam and Eve were spiritually dead, yet their minds were so conditioned to God that it was easy to hear from Him. Even their children grew up in an environment where the knowledge of God was still so real that they too, were tuned into the frequency of heaven. Where does this leave us?

It is my desire to reveal to you God's ever supporting presence so that you will boldly manifest His ability with regularity. Developing an awareness of Him at all times is such an essential key to continued spiritual success; confirmed in signs and wonders.

As I believe you can now understand, it is possible that even with our salvation in place, and being right with God on every count, we often are so conditioned by the mind of the world that we are insensitive to all God is and all that He wants to do in and through us. Do you see why renewing the mind, meditation and, if you will, washing the mind clean from the filth of the world's mentalities and suggestions is so important?

If the church knows what they possess in Christ, their rights and privileges, and yet they still are not seeing the miraculous evidence of the supernatural, there can be but one answer. **We are not sure that God will do what He said.**

Without a healthy expectation of what God will do faith has no real action. Get ready to develop the mind of Christ. Be prepared to receive the faith and confidence to be continually aware of His presence and walk in His power. God's nature and way of doing things will become so natural to you that the supernatural in your life will become as natural as breathing and walking!

Keys to Living in the Miraculous

- Be continually aware of God's presence.

- Don't put God into your box.

- Be renewed in your mind so that you can *think right.*

- Embrace the mind of Christ.

- Expect the aroma of His presence to continually saturate you.

- Understand that you have been restored to "His image" as a new creation able to hear His voice and know His ways.

- Realize and believe that God *is able to do* exceedingly abundantly, beyond all that you can think or imagine!

Chapter 2

EXPECTATION BIRTHS MIRACLES

FAITH, HOPE AND LOVE ARE THREE forces that God recognizes in the earth as essential. Paul wrote, "And now these three remain: faith, hope and love. But the greatest of these is love" (1 Cor. 13:13 NIV). For years now, hope has been disparaged and devalued. Any one holding fast to faith has been warned about hope. Hope has been dismissed as with the attitude: *those who just hope will never see anything happen.* Yet, Paul inspired by the Holy Ghost mentions hope as necessary and essential in our Christian walk.

In Greek, hope (*elpis*) means "expectation, whether of good or of ill." Rarely does hope expect evil or fear the future. Most often, hope is the "expectation of good, hope; and in the Christian sense, joyful and **confident expectation** of eternal salvation: Acts

23:6." (From *Thayer's Greek Lexicon, Electronic Database* by Biblesoft).

Notice the terminology of the bold print: a **confident expectation** with a joyful attitude. The *Strong's Concordance* also adds, "anticipation with pleasure." This certainly sounds different than the worldly understanding of hope. Usually we see hope as a nice thought that most likely will never come true. Kind of like Walt Disney's Jiminy Cricket who sings, "When you wish upon a star...." Hope is seen as wishful thinking, "it sure would be nice if it happened, but I'm sure it won't."

Hope defined as wishful certainly does not prepare for success. On the contrary, there is preparation for the worst. This sounds like Mr. Murphy's Law, "If something bad is going to happen, it will probably happen to me." With this mentality, anyone would feel like the circumstances of life and the cards that have been dealt to one govern life. Such thinking embraces a fatalistic view of the future with a life strategy of making a good defense one's offence.

The biblical view of hope is much different than the world's view. Faith heroes in Scripture refuse to sit back with the attitude: "Let's see what might happen." Or, "Maybe my wishes will come true." The beauty about faith is that we have God's answer before we approach the problems of life. Faith is the assurance of things hoped for! Having such assurance, how does confident expectation birth miracles?

The Substance of Hope

Hebrews 11:1 declares, "Now faith is the substance of things hoped for, the evidence of things not seen." Let's repeat this verse with the definition of hope added. "Now faith is the substance of things **confidently expected**, the evidence of things not seen."

Faith in God through Christ fills hope with substance and becomes the evidence when what you expect is not immediately seen. Understand that there is a natural desire or hope for things to happen in life. For example, the moment you feel sick, there is a desire for the sickness to leave. No one ever exclaims, "How wonderful, I'm getting sick." Because God did not create you to experience sickness, pain, depression, poverty and oppression, you revolt immediately and desire change. This is natural hope. This hope is not filled with a concrete solution.

People become hopeless when all natural remedies have been applied, and there remains no change. Just a casual reading of the Bible brings you to the conclusion that worldly hope is not God's way of life. The Bible simplified is God's plan for man. God desires to be involved in every aspect of our lives until the advan-tage of the **Holy Spirit** swallows up the natural.

God is the *God of hope*. Rom 15:13 proclaims, "May the God of hope fill you with all joy and peace as you trust in him, so that you may overflow with hope by the power of the Holy Spirit" (NIV). Guaranteed, you cannot act in effective faith, without confidently expecting in God who is the author of all expectations.

Living In The Miraculous

In 1994 my wife, Erin, and I received a word from the Lord to have our first child. We were traveling at the time with the Rhema Singers and Band. At this time with the group, having a child would most likely cause you to leave the road. So, the Lord instructed us to have our first child. We learned that we were expecting in June.

Nine months away would put the baby's due date around March. Outside of the test result that my wife was pregnant, I couldn't tell any difference. My expectations were not full; timing has a great deal to do with one's expectations. Also, the amount of evidence you have plays a big part. As you can imagine, the individual who has great evidence in the courtroom has the most confidence in the outcome. During the beginning weeks, I would forget many times that we were going to have a baby. It seemed so far off, and there wasn't any change in our lives.

Suddenly toward the end of the third month there seemed to be a little evidence. As time progressed, the evidence became more substantial that we were going to have a baby. When you see a woman who looks pregnant, you say that she is expecting. The greater the evidence the more moved you are to make preparations. As mentioned earlier, timing has much to do with the force of expectancy.

For instance, I'm not going to rush my wife to the hospital in the third month for the delivery of our child. Why not? Because she is not due! However, when her due date arrived, we had a bag already packed. Can you see how important expectancy is to the manifestation?

Hope Prompts Faith to Act

John writes about this kind of expectant hope. "Behold what manner of love the Father has bestowed on us, that we should be called children of God! Therefore the world does not know us, because it did not know Him. Beloved, now we are children of God; and it has not yet been revealed what we shall be, but we know that when He is revealed, we shall be like Him, for we shall see Him as He is. And everyone who has this hope in Him purifies himself, just as He is pure" (1 John 3:1-3).

As you read this scripture, you can see that faith and hope work together. In verse two there is need of a revelation of the children of God. What is it that we know? We know that we are children of God. We know that He shall be revealed. We know that we shall be like Him. We also know that we shall see Him as He is. Remember, James said that without the action of faith, faith is dead, or without profit.

The action of our belief stated above is to purify ourselves just as He is pure. Now here is where timing comes in again. If Jesus were coming tomorrow, there would be a great emphasis placed on purity. This verse of scripture is becoming a real factor today because of the signs of His coming. Two months before my wife and I left the road with Brother Hagin to work in Prayer and Healing School I had an experience with expectancy and action that definitely made an impression.

We had just come home from a Holy Ghost meeting with Brother Hagin to our new home. We had only been in that home for a couple of weeks. We had signed the paper for the home, moved our things in and then a couple of days later went on the road for two weeks. We were glad to get home.

The phone rang and I answered it. The man on the other end of the phone with a rough voice introduced himself as the IRS. It was Brother Hagin trying to play a joke on me. I recognized him right away and then he asked me what we were doing. I told him not much and then asked him the same question. He said that he and Mrs. Hagin (mom) were coming over to see our new house. I asked him when he was coming, he said, right now.

When Erin asked who it was and what they wanted I told her that Mom and Dad Hagin wanted to come over to see our house. She asked when and I told her "They're on the way." Immediately she began to check around the house to make sure everything was in place.

You may laugh at what I did, although it was influenced by something Brother Hagin preached in the meeting we were just in. He told the story of the days when he and his wife used to travel, before it was common to stay in hotels. Most traveling ministers would stay in the homes of the pastors. He commented that when stepping inside a home that he was to stay in, he and his wife could usually pick up on the spiritual climate of the home.

For instance, whether or not there was strife and contentions, or if harsh words were spoken. For some reason, when Brother Hagin said that they were coming over, and that they were on the way, that was the first thing that came to mind. So while Erin was tidying up a few things, I went into every room of our house, and quietly said, "I love my wife." Just in case I had said something I shouldn't and forgot to apologize, I was making sure there were plenty of loving words in our home.

Now, you may be enjoying this from a humorous point of view, however, it does illustrate well how expectancy works with time. If Brother Hagin said that he was coming over a year from next Saturday, would we have been so quickly moved to act as we did? Of course not! The anticipation of them being there at any time produced an urgency to act.

Faith Acts on Hope—Confident Expectation

Now concerning redemption, when was this great work accomplished for us? We know according to Paul, "that God was in Christ, reconciling the whole world unto Himself" (2 Cor. 5:19). Two thousand years ago, freedom over all the works of the devil was placed on your record. The world needs to hear that God is in love with them and has already made provision for their freedom. You received this wonderful gift by believing in your heart that God raised Jesus from the dead, and confessing Jesus as your Lord.

This is a great truth that should be cause for great excitement because everything necessary for the experience of your salvation has been given to you. Paul said that we have been given all things that pertain to life and godliness. So my question would be, "How long do you have to wait for your healing?"

Isaiah declared that Jesus took our infirmities and bore our pains and that with His stripes we are healed (Read Isaiah 53:3-5). If this is already done, then what are we waiting on? If we have to wait for it to happen, we then can't act until we're sure it has. Isaiah describes best what faith coupled with expectant confidence is:

> *Have you not known?*
> *Have you not heard?*
> *The everlasting God, the LORD,*
> *The Creator of the ends of the earth,*
> *Neither faints nor is weary.*
> *His understanding is unsearchable.*
>
> *He gives power to the weak,*
> *And to those who have no might He*
>   *increases strength.*
> *Even the youths shall faint and be weary,*
> *And the young men shall utterly fall,*
> *But those who wait on the LORD*
> *Shall renew their strength;*
> *They shall mount up with wings like eagles,*

They shall run and not be weary,
They shall walk and not faint. (Isa. 40:28-31)

What we know for certain is that God neither faints nor is weary. Also, He gives power to the weak, and increases strength to those who have none. Naturally youth will faint and be weary and young men will fall; yet God wants you to know that there is supernatural assistance for His people. Where the world fails, the believer succeeds; where weakness is present, strength abounds.

Even though sickness, pain, poverty and lack try to come to every person in this cursed world, we are not cursed but blessed. The knowledge that God gives strength is what causes you to wait on the Lord. You may be thinking, "I thought we were not waiting on redemption realities?" That is absolutely true.

The word *wait* in this verse doesn't mean what you think. It means "to expect." They that *expect* in the Lord shall renew their strength. Your expectancy works with your faith in God as the giver of strength.

In Isaiah 40:31, we read that two things happen when we expect the Lord to give us strength. One is strength is renewed and the other is mounting up with wings as eagles. Let me ask a question at this point, was the spirit world here first or this natural world?

Very easily you would answer, "The spirit world." Hebrews 11:3 tells us that God created the visible by the invisible. So in verse 31 the strength and ability to mount up with the wings, as an eagle, is God's spiritual endowment and answer to your need. You may be thinking it would be a whole lot easier if God just took the weariness away. **If sickness or weariness comes and goes on its own, then you don't control it. It controls you.**

However, if in response to your acceptance of God's ability you possess a spiritual solution, then you are in the driver's seat. Yes, but my body still feels weary you may protest. This is the very reason why faith and hope work so well together. If you have God's answer for your weariness even though your body still feels weary, you can run because you know you have the answer. And, with expectant confidence, you will act in faith on God's Word—not being weary, and then weariness leaves.

We know that the easiest and most rational thing to do when you feel faint is to lie down and rest until the faintness leaves, right? According to verse 31, if you know that God is the supplier of strength and you have willingly received it by faith, even though your body may still have the symptoms, you expect them to leave you as you act well because you are which means you will walk and then not be faint. Wow, does this sound different than the world's way of doing things?

This may even sound different than the faith teaching you've received. Especially if you're confessing that you believe you received, but you're waiting on the manifestation. It would seem here, as the Bible points out, that your manifestation is waiting on you. We will cover this thought further in a later chapter.

Here's what I want you to understand: **Continually expect from God and constantly act on the Word.**

If you have little or no expectancy in your life, it's in direct proportion to the evidence of the Word that has inspired your faith. You may say, "Well, I'm expecting from God." Are you doing what you couldn't do? If you're not, then what are you expect-ing? Remember something profound that Jesus said in John 5:24, "He that believeth, hath."

Or you could say, when you believe, you have the answer. Which means the answer replaced the prob-lem, right? So, why wouldn't the answer work? If you bought a new car, yet never drove it, wouldn't that be strange? If someone questioned you about it and you replied, "The reason I haven't driven it yet is because I don't expect it to work." Then why did you buy it? Do you see what is being said? Why do we trust God if we don't expect there to be change. Why would I wait to see change if I received the answer?

For example, if someone wired money to my account and the bank called me to confirm that it was there, would I have a problem writing a check? Of course not. However, if you think about it, I didn't see the money. Well, you'd say, but the bank called you and told you it was there. And so they did. Did God ever call you and tell you that healing, money, peace, joy, and many other blessings were there? You've received hundreds of phone calls, confirming that your account is full. God daily loads you with benefits and every spiritual blessing is yours.

Is it possible that these thoughts could cause you to expect change? Would the action of your faith be the natural response to your confident expectation? Someone should shout, maybe run around the room, dance, jump up and down or at least have a party or celebration. Thank God, I'm expecting miracles in my life, how about you?

I want to express to you as strongly as I can, just how important the first two chapters of this book are. I would suggest reading them again before going on. When you understand just how poisoned our minds have been from the world's way of thinking, you will consciously renew your mind with the Word of God. As you see the difference between saying that you expect God to do for you and acting on the Word because you do expect, your thinking will be challenged in many areas of your life.

From this point on, I will give you evidence from the Bible that God will do what He says He will do. At any point in the reading of the following chapters, you can receive your miracle. Remember, this material is not just to inspire you to receive what you need, really salvation took care of that, but you should also be inspired and encouraged to minister to others.

Keys to Living in the Miraculous

- Know that hope means much more than "wish;" it means "confident expectation."
- Let hope prompt your faith to act.

- Act in confident, expectant faith to see the invisible manifested.

- Stop waiting for a manifestation, act in hope to walk into your manifestation.

- Wait...that means *expect* God to renew your strength.

- Act on your expectation that God will do what He says He will do.

- Expect to receive your miracle.

- Begin to minister to others in expectant confidence, i.e. hope.

Chapter 3

IN THE BEGINNING, GOD!

"IN THE BEGINNING GOD CREATED THE heavens and the earth" (Gen. 1:1). In order to understand more the mind of God, it's best to see God from God's perspective. God revealed many names for Himself through which He describes His different attributes and characteristics.

In the first verse of the Bible, God reveals His name as *Elohim*. *Elohim* is the Hebrew for the one, true and only God. I ask you to look closely at the **bold** words in Genesis 1 and a few verses in Genesis 2.

> In the beginning **God** created the heavens and the earth. The earth was without form, and void; and darkness was on the face of the deep. And the Spirit of God was hovering over the face of the waters. Then **God** said,

"Let there be light"; and there was light. And **God** saw the light, that it was good; and **God** divided the light from the darkness. **God** called the light Day, and the darkness He called Night. So the evening and the morning were the first day.

Then **God** said, "Let there be a firmament in the midst of the waters, and let it divide the waters from the waters." Thus **God** made the firmament, and divided the waters which were under the firmament from the waters which were above the firmament; and it was so. And **God** called the firmament Heaven. So the evening and the morning were the second day.

Then **God** said, "Let the waters under the heavens be gathered together into one place, and let the dry land appear"; and it was so. And **God** called the dry land Earth, and the gathering together of the waters He called Seas. And **God** saw that it was good. Then **God** said, "Let the earth bring forth grass, the herb that yields seed, and the fruit tree that yields fruit according to its kind, whose seed is in itself, on the earth"; and it was so. And the earth brought forth grass, the herb that yields seed according to its kind, and the tree that yields fruit, whose seed is in itself according to its kind. And **God** saw that it was good. So the evening and the morning were the third day.

*Then **God** said, "Let there be lights in the firmament of the heavens to divide the day from the night; and let them be for signs and seasons, and for days and years; and let them be for lights in the firmament of the heavens to give light on the earth"; and it was so. Then **God** made two great lights: the greater light to rule the day, and the lesser light to rule the night. He made the stars also. **God** set them in the firmament of the heavens to give light on the earth, and to rule over the day and over the night, and to divide the light from the darkness. And **God** saw that it was good. So the evening and the morning were the fourth day.*

*Then **God** said, "Let the waters abound with an abundance of living creatures, and let birds fly above the earth across the face of the firmament of the heavens." So **God** created great sea creatures and every living thing that moves, with which the waters abounded, according to their kind, and every winged bird according to its kind. And **God** saw that it was good. And **God** blessed them, saying, "Be fruitful and multiply, and fill the waters in the seas, and let birds multiply on the earth." So the evening and the morning were the fifth day.*

*Then **God** said, "Let the earth bring forth the living creature according to its kind: cattle and creeping thing and beast of the* earth, each according to its kind"; and it was so. And **God** made the beast of the earth according to its kind, cattle according to its kind, and everything that creeps on the earth according to its kind. And **God** saw that it was good.

Then **God** said, "Let Us make man in Our image, according to Our likeness; let them have dominion over the fish of the sea, over the birds of the air, and over the cattle, over all the earth and over every creeping thing that creeps on the earth." So **God** created man in His own image; in the image of **God** He created him; male and female He created them. Then **God** blessed them, and **God** said to them, "Be fruitful and multiply; fill the earth and subdue it; have dominion over the fish of the sea, over the birds of the air, and over every living thing that moves on the earth."

And **God** said, "See, I have given you every herb that yields seed which is on the face of all the earth, and every tree whose fruit yields seed; to you it shall be for food. Also, to every beast of the earth, to every bird of the air, and to everything that creeps on the earth, in which there is life, I have given every green herb for food"; and it was so. Then **God** saw everything that He had made, and indeed it was very good. So the evening and the morning were the sixth day.

> *Thus the heavens and the earth, and all the host of them, were finished. And on the seventh day **God** ended His work which He had done, and He rested on the seventh day from all His work which He had done. Then **God** blessed the seventh day and sanctified it, because in it He rested from all His work which **God** had created and made.*
>
> *This is the history of the heavens and the earth when they were created, in the day that the **LORD God** made the earth and the heavens.*

As you can see from chapter one to chapter two the highlighted words are **God**. Is it as interesting to you as to me that the fourth verse of chapter two stands out as different from all the rest? It's kind of like the games they have for children, where you find the picture that is different from all the rest. The name Elohim is used for 31 verses of the first chapter and 3 verses of the second chapter before another name for God is introduced.

The God Who Reveals Himself

I believe the significance must be found in the meaning of the name. The word **LORD God** is (*Yahweh-Elohim* or *Jehovah-Elohim*) in the Hebrew, which means, the self-existent one who reveals Himself. We understand that no one created God. He has always been and always will be. He is self-existent. Lord also means He reveals Himself. The word *reveal* could be stated, manifests, discloses, declare and to show.

There is a compounded significance to the word Jehovah that is very important. God has chosen to use this word in conjunction with covenants. Wherever you see the word Jehovah, the way God reveals Himself, is in the form of covenant with His people forever. One way to validate the use of Jehovah is to see if Jesus in the New Testament has fulfilled in His earth walk the meaning of the word used in the Old Testament. Connect the two words together (Jehovah and *Elohim*) and their meaning by defini-tion would be, **"The Self Existent One who Reveals Himself as The One and Only True God."**

I believe a good illustration will help you understand the significance of this definition being placed in verse four after creation had been completed. Erin and I have been blessed with three children, all girls. My oldest daughter is Alli, in the middle is Drew and our youngest is Chloe. All three are wonderful. We love them dearly. If you have children you will understand what I'm about to say, and if not you can surely imagine.

It is such a thrill to see your children born into the world. Each child being born is equally exciting; however, the first birth is unique because as parents it's a new experience for you. When Alli came into the world, I remember how beautiful she was. The nurses cleaned her and wrapped her up in a blanket and handed her to me. Wow!

On one hand, I didn't know what to do; yet on the

other hand it was so natural to hold her. I walked a few feet away from all that was going on as the doctors were helping Erin and said softly to Alli, "I'm your daddy. Before God I make a commitment to take care of you all the days of your life. You will always have the best. You will never lack for food, clothing, strength or health. You will grow up to know Jesus as your Lord and Savior." (I may regret that one about the clothing one of these days, especially with three girls.)

Think back to the reason why God used a different name once creation had been completed. There was no reason to use the name Jehovah in Genesis 1:1 was there? There would have been no one to receive the revelation. When everything was just right, God stepped out in plain view of all creation, especially man, and revealed, declared and showed Himself as their Daddy. Can you imagine all creation looking up and beholding God's awesomeness and hearing Him say, "I am Jehovah *Elohim*. I make an everlasting covenant with you, that I am the one and only true God who made all that is. From this day, you are forever taken care of, all is yours to enjoy. As the one and only true God you will never need to honor another."

If you think about it, God's revelation to Adam and Eve was all that was necessary to resist the temptations of the devil. That is why the first of the Ten Commandments is, *there shall be no other god's before Me.*

Was Jesus a fulfillment of this covenant? John 14:6 says, "I am the way, the truth, and the life, no man comes to the Father but by me." Jesus was and is the one and only true God. Does your heart leap within you? God didn't just play a tape recorder with the words quoted above, He became visible in Jesus Christ. God actually revealed Himself. All creation beheld Him and listened to His declaration.

At the beginning of history, there was no reason for God to reveal Himself in any other way. He didn't need to reveal Himself as healer, because no one was sick. The main point of this discussion is that God wants to be seen. Paul tells us in Eph 2:6-7, "...and raised us up together, and made us sit together in the heavenly places in Christ Jesus, that in the ages to come He might show the exceeding riches of His grace in His kindness toward us in Christ Jesus."

Just like the beginning of all things, God stays true to character. In the end, God is going to put on a show for all eternity. I believe throughout all eternity, God will never exhaust His vastness. There will be a new side of God revealed to us every day forever. I don't think we will ever stop expressing awe.

Jehovah Does What He Promises From Beginning to End!

If God is Alpha and Omega then He is everything in between. As we study briefly the call and ministry of Moses we will see the willingness of God to reveal Himself to His people. When God originally revealed Himself to His creation, He was establishing a precedent for all times. Never will you find God unwilling to manifest to His people His goodness, character and love. Let's look at how God called Moses to the ministry.

> *Now Moses was tending the flock of Jethro his father-in-law, the priest of Midian, and he led the flock to the far side of the desert and came to Horeb, the mountain of God. There the angel of the LORD appeared to him in flames of fire from within a bush. Moses saw that though the bush was on fire it did not burn up. So Moses thought, "I will go over and see this strange sight—why the bush does not burn up."* (Exodus 3:1-3 NIV)

From the beginning, God called Moses with the supernatural. Does this seem to fit the personality of Jehovah? Of course it does. God is revealing Himself to Moses. Throughout the dialogue that follows, God convinces Moses to accept the responsibility to deliver the people of Israel. Moses begins to question God as to how he is going to convince Israel to follow him and Pharaoh to obey him.

> *"Go, assemble the elders of Israel and say to them, 'The LORD, the God of your fathers— the God of Abraham, Isaac and Jacob— appeared to me and said: I have watched over you and have seen what has been done to you in Egypt. And I have promised to*

bring you up out of your misery in Egypt into the land of the Canaanites, Hittites, Amorites, Perizzites, Hivites and Jebusites—a land flowing with milk and honey.'

"The elders of Israel will listen to you. Then you and the elders are to go to the king of Egypt and say to him, 'The LORD, the God of the Hebrews, has met with us. Let us take a three-day journey into the desert to offer sacrifices to the LORD our God.' But I know that the king of Egypt will not let you go unless a mighty hand compels him. So I will stretch out my hand and strike the Egyptians with all the wonders that I will perform among them. After that, he will let you go.

"And I will make the Egyptians favorably disposed toward this people, so that when you leave you will not go empty-handed. Every woman is to ask her neighbor and any woman living in her house for articles of silver and gold and for clothing, which you will put on your sons and daughters. And so you will plunder the Egyptians."

Moses answered, "What if they do not believe me or listen to me and say, 'The LORD did not appear to you'?" (Exodus 3:16-4:1 NIV)

Remember, God is training Moses to think like Him. Moses will learn to expect God to miraculously back him up. Likewise, God is endeavoring through these examples to encourage us to see things from His perspective. I can hear some saying, "Because they didn't have the word, they needed the miraculous."

This is the same mentality that so many have concerning missionary work. Erroneously people think that God has to show up with power in heathen countries so that people will believe the Word. The real truth concerning missionary work is that people who don't know any better simply believe what you tell them God will do. More miracles happen because of simple faith in the gospel message about Jesus than any other way.

When we preach God's life changing message, He will back it up with all kinds of signs and wonders. Remember, God shows up because He by His nature is the God who reveals Himself. God is a bottom line God. Even though people are at different levels of maturity and development, every life should display the miraculous of God.

Jehovah Desires to Do the Miraculous in Your Life!

The following verses continue to build a case for us to expect God to work with us to gain confidence in His desire to reveal Himself.

> Then the LORD said to him, "What is that in your hand?"
> "A staff," he replied.

> The LORD said, "Throw it on the ground."
>
> Moses threw it on the ground and it became a snake, and he ran from it. Then the LORD said to him, "Reach out your hand and take it by the tail." So Moses reached out and took hold of the snake and it turned back into a staff in his hand. "This," said the LORD, "is so that they may believe that the LORD, the God of their fathers—the God of Abraham, the God of Isaac and the God of Jacob—has appeared to you."
>
> Then the LORD said, "Put your hand inside your cloak." So Moses put his hand into his cloak, and when he took it out, it was leprous, like snow.
>
> "Now put it back into your cloak," he said. So Moses put his hand back into his cloak, and when he took it out, it was restored, like the rest of his flesh.
>
> Then the LORD said, "If they do not believe you or pay attention to the first miraculous sign, they may believe the second. But if they do not believe these two signs or listen to you, take some water from the Nile and pour it on the dry ground. The water you take from the river will become blood on the ground." (Exodus 4:2-9 NIV)

Before God called Moses there was a burning bush. To settle and secure Moses in the assignment on his life, there are two more miracles. In these same miracles Moses is instructed to use as proof to the people and Pharaoh that God is with him.

This mentality that you are seeing has Jehovah written all over it. I can still hear people saying, "Well we have the word today, we don't need these signs and wonders." Think of what that statement means, "We have the word." That's awesome. The Word of God is a written manifest of what you can expect God to do. It's the reason why we as faith people are to bring the miraculous into every day life.

In Exodus 6 the Lord says something to Moses that makes the whole story very interesting.

> *Then the LORD said to Moses, "Now you will see what I will do to Pharaoh: Because of my mighty hand he will let them go; because of my mighty hand he will drive them out of his country."*
>
> *God also said to Moses, "I am the LORD. I appeared to Abraham, to Isaac and to Jacob as God Almighty, but by my name the LORD I did not make myself known to them. I also established my covenant with them to give them the land of Canaan, where they lived as aliens. Moreover, I have heard the groaning of the Israelites, whom the Egyptians are enslaving, and I have remembered my covenant.*
>
> *"Therefore, say to the Israelites: 'I am the LORD, and I will bring you out from under the yoke of the Egyptians. I will free you from being slaves to them, and I will redeem*

you with an outstretched arm and with mighty acts of judgment. I will take you as my own people, and I will be your God. Then you will know that I am the LORD your God, who brought you out from under the yoke of the Egyptians. And I will bring you to the land I swore with uplifted hand to give to Abraham, to Isaac and to Jacob. I will give it to you as a possession. I am the LORD.'" (Exodus 6:1-8 NIV)

In verse two God says that *I am the Lord, or Jehovah,* the God who reveals Himself. Notice He said that He appeared to Abraham, to Isaac and to Jacob as God Almighty, signifying God's power and dominion. He said that He didn't make Himself known as Jehovah or revealer. This thought will be the cause for the discussion in the next chapter.

Do you see how God is revealing Himself to Moses? God is making it plain that from the very conception of the call on Moses' life for this assignment, to the completion of the assignment, there will be much revelation and manifestation.

This sounds like a dream come true for the modern believer. Maybe it is the reason for the Apostle Paul spending so much of his time praying for the church to have a spirit of wisdom and revelation in the knowledge of God.

If people could just see, understand and believe the availability of God's power and God's desire for that ability to be used, there

would then be greater displays of God in our midst. Zephaniah 3:17 says that the Lord our God in the midst of us is mighty. Is He just mighty to be mighty, or is He mighty for a purpose? Wouldn't it seem that God is mighty to do the things that need something powerful to make them Godly?

In the life of Moses with his assignment to deliver the children of Israel, the supernatural played such a huge role in their deliverance. The supernatural played a tremendous role in your deliverance too. It took you from darkness into the love and light of God's eternal kingdom. You became a new creature in a moment of time.

You had a miracle birth and entered into a miracle existence. As theologians will tell you, the miracle deliverance of the children of Israel represents our new birth. The possession of the Promised Land is the life lived by the believer.

Jehovah is the beginning and the end. Jehovah is the God who reveals and shows up not just for Moses but also for you! Jehovah is there at the beginning of your new life in Christ and continues to reveal Himself throughout your whole life as *the God* who will do the miraculous for you just as with the children of Israel. They were delivered from slavery into the Promised Land experiencing miracle after miracle.

The same God, Jehovah, who did the miraculous in their lives is ready to act supernaturally in your life. You can expect Jehovah's miracles today!

Keys to Living in the Miraculous

- God your Creator (*Elohim*) still creates today.

- Jehovah (*Yahweh*) God (*Elohim*) is still revealing Himself today to those who trust in Jesus Christ.

- Jehovah God reveals Himself in miracles, signs and wonders today just as He did to Moses and the children of Israel thousands of years ago.

- Are you expecting Jehovah God to be Himself in your life? To fill your life daily from beginning to end with the miraculous?

- The same Jehovah God of Moses lives today and you can expect Him to be true to His Nature—to reveal Himself in signs and wonders!

Chapter 4

FAITH ACTS ON GOD'S COVENANT PROMISES

B<small>UT A<small>BRAM</small> SAID</small>, *"*L<small>ORD</small> GOD, *what will you give me, seeing I go childless, and the heir of my house is Eliezer of Damascus?"* (Genesis 15:2)

Abram questioned the living God on a promise that God has made. Is that faith?

In Genesis 12 God unequivocally promised to Abram His future plan. This plan included having a son through whom all the nations of the earth would be blessed. In Genesis 15, Abram begins to question the lack of evidence to the promise given. Asking questions of God is not wrong; it's how we learn.

However, when it's time to operate in faith and believe God, your questions should be answered by the Word of God. Faith is always inspired by the Word of God. The reason why it's so exciting to believe the Word of God is that God has predetermined the outcome. Our success is already secure.

Believing God is relying on a greater evidence—the Word of God— than the present circumstances.

God immediately moved Abram into faith by insuring him that what He has previously promised him will come to pass. Genesis 15:5 reads, "Then He brought him outside and said, "Look now toward heaven, and count the stars if you are able to number them." And He said to him, "So shall your descendants be." God used something very common to Abram to encourage his faith. Abram had been raised in a culture that worshipped the moon. He was used to looking at the stars. God made a simple adjustment with Abram and immediately in that area Abram believed.

The next verse says just that, "And he believed in the LORD, and He accounted it to him for righteousness" (Gen. 15:6). With that settled, God began to speak to Abram about the land that He promised to Abram, "Then He said to him, 'I am the LORD, who brought you out of Ur of the Chaldeans, to give you this land to inherit it'" (Gen. 15:7). God has already promised him this land; in fact Abram is already occupying the land. Abram is having problems believing God. He is to us through the New Testament the father of faith; however, he didn't start there.

The Immutable Power of Blood Covenant

God did something very radical for Abram that caused Abram to become very radical in his believing. In verse 8 Abram said, "Lord GOD, how shall I know that I will inherit it?" So God said to him, "Bring Me a three-year-old heifer, a three-year-old female goat, a three-year-old ram, a turtledove, and a young pigeon." To many people today, this response is very foreign. Why would God answer Abram by telling him to seek out and bring a three-year-old heifer, a three-year-old female goat, a three-year-old ram, a turtledove, and a young pigeon?

But in Abram's culture, he was familiar with animal sacrifice. So we read, "Then he brought all these to Him and cut them in two, down the middle, and placed each piece opposite the other; but he did not cut the birds in two" (Gen. 15:10). The reason why I know that Abram knew what to do is because he made preparations for the sacrifice before his instructions to do so. Really, all God asked Abram to do was to bring the animals and birds.

Abram prepared the animals for a sacrifice. The preparation that Abram made is distinctly made for a blood sacrifice. This ceremony cuts the animals down the middle and places them opposite the other. Again, God was willing to answer Abram's questions with something that was easy for Abram to comprehend, thereby securing Abram's trust in the midst of questioning.

We will see from this blood covenant that God not only put in motion the redemption of mankind,

He also eliminated doubt from Abram's mind concerning anything that God revealed or promised to him. This last statement alone is profound. Is it really possible that a ceremony could eliminate doubt from a person's conscience concerning anything spoken there after?

The fact that this statement is true is a testament to the power of a blood covenant. Of course, if you have no revelation of the ritual, the impact would not be the same. This is one of the greatest reasons why the church does not move in the power of God. There is very little respect for the Word of God, for covenant, or for the shedding of blood. Once covenant is established, Abram knew that the word of your covenant partner was his bond. Abram *knew* that God would be bound by both His Word and His covenant to do exactly as He had promised. Of course, God also had the omnipotent power to accomplish whatever He covenanted to do no matter how impossible that covenant promise was to man. Obviously, God is the ultimate partner.

Hebrews six will help us understand this covenant in light of Jehovah the God who reveals Himself.

> *For when God made a promise to Abraham, because He could swear by no one greater, He swore by Himself, saying, "Surely blessing I will bless you, and multiplying I will multiply you." And so, after he had patiently endured, he obtained the promise. For men indeed swear by the greater, and an oath for*

confirmation is for them an end of all dispute. Thus God, determining to show more abundantly to the heirs of promise the immutability of His counsel, confirmed it by an oath, that by two immutable things, in which it is impossible for God to lie, we might have strong consolation, who have fled for refuge to lay hold of the hope set before us. This hope we have as an anchor of the soul, both sure and steadfast, and which enters the Presence behind the veil, where the forerunner has entered for us, even Jesus, having become High Priest forever according to the order of Melchizedek. (Heb. 6:13-20)

The Significance of Blood Covenant for the Miraculous

In a blood covenant you would always seek out one greater than yourself with whom to cut a covenant. It is always to your advantage to find someone more prosperous, stronger in battle and in every way greater than you to enter into covenant with. The significance of the blood covenant is that it is a complete merging of two lives into one.

You lose your identity as you knew it when you commit your life to another. Life is no longer only about what you want; you must consider your partner. There is a very serious side to this commitment. To explain further and in detail I want to quote from

The Miracle of the Scarlet Thread, pages 28-31, "When two Hebrew males entered into a blood covenant they went through a very specific ceremony."

To explain this to you, I want to give you an example of what might happen if you and I entered into a blood covenant as two Hebrew males would do it. There are nine steps from *The Miracle of the Scarlet Thread* that I have adapted for you here:

Step 1—Take Off Coat or Robe

My first act would be to take off my coat or robe and give it to you. Now to the Hebrew, a person's robe represents the person. By taking off my robe and giving it to you, I'm symbolically saying, "I'm giving you all myself. My total being and my life, I pledge to you." And then you would do the same to me.

Step 2—Take Off a Belt

Next, I take off my belt and give it to you. Now I don't use my belt to hold up my pants, but to hold up my weapons. My belt holds my armor together; my dagger, my bow and arrow, my sword. So symbolically I'm giving you all my strength and pledging you all my support and protection. And as I give you my belt, I'm saying, "Here is my strength and all my ability to fight. If anybody attacks you, they are also attacking me. Your battles are my battles and mine are yours. I will fight with you. I will help defend you and protect you."

And you do the same to me. This is similar to a compact nations might make today. But this one cannot be broken.

Step 3—Cut the Covenant

The next step is to actually "cut the covenant" by taking an animal and splitting it right down the middle. In the Bible, an animal is only cut down the middle and split in two in a covenant ceremony.

After we split the animal, we lay each half to the side of us and stand in between the two bloody halves of flesh, with our backs to each other. Then we walk right through the bloody halves, making a figure eight, and come back to face each other.

In doing so we are saying two things. First, we are saying that we are dying to ourselves, giving up the rights to our own life and beginning a new walk with our covenant partner unto death. You see, in this covenant, each half of the dead animal represents us.

Second, since the blood covenant is the most solemn pact, we each point down to the bloody animal split in two and say, "God do so to me and more if I ever try to break this covenant. Just split me right down the middle and feed me to the vultures because I tried to break the most sacred of all compacts."

Step 4—Raise the Right Arm and Mix Blood

Then we raise our right arms, cut our palms and bring them together. As we do, our blood intermingles. Then we swear allegiance to each other.

Remember how you did that as a kid? With eyes probably half closed, you and your closest friend pricked your finger and brought them together swearing allegiance forever until mom broke the covenant for you.

As our blood intermingles, we believe our lives are intermingling and becoming one life. This is because our blood is our life and to intermingle blood is to intermingle life.

So we are putting off our old nature and putting on the nature of our blood covenant partner. We two are becoming one. Man has always believed that intermingling blood is intermingling life. This symbolically shows the two of us becoming one.

Step 5—Exchange Names

Then as we stand there with our blood intermingling, we exchange names. I take your last name as part of my name, and you take my last name as part of your name.

Step 6—Make a Scar

The next step is to rub our blood together and make a scar as a permanent testimony to the covenant. The scar will bear witness to the covenant we have made. It will always be there to remind us of our covenant responsibilities to each other. It is the guarantee of our covenant.

If anyone tries to harm us, all we have to do is raise up that right arm and show our scar. By that we are saying, "There's more to me than meets the eye. If you're coming after me, you're also going to have to fight my blood covenant partner. And you don't know how big he is. So what are you going to do? Are you going to take your chances or back off? If the would be attacker has any sense, he's going to back off. So the scar is our seal that testifies to the covenant.

Henry Stanley, on his explorations through Africa, cut covenant fifty times with various chieftains. And we can certainly understand why. Anytime he would come across an unfriendly tribe, he would just hold up that right arm with those fifty scars and any would be attacker would take off running in the other direction.

Today, when we meet friends, we don't show scars, we shake hands. There are many trappings of blood covenant in our modern society; we've just eliminated the blood.

Step 7—Give Covenant Terms

Then we stand before witnesses and give the terms of the covenant. I say, "All my assets are yours. All my money, all my property and all my possessions are yours. If you need any of them, you don't even have to ask. Just come and get it. What's mine is yours and what's yours is mine. And if I die, all my children are yours by adoption and you are responsible for my family.

But at the same time, you also get my liabilities. If I ever get in trouble financially, I don't come ask you for money. I come to you and say, "Where's our checkbook?"

We are in covenant. Everything I have is yours and yours is mine, both assets and liabilities. So we stand there and read off, before witnesses, our list of assets and liabilities.

Step 8—Eat a Memorial Meal

Then we have a memorial meal to complete the covenant union. In place of the animal and blood, we have bread and wine. In the Bible, wine is called the blood of the grapes (Genesis 49:11) and it represents our own lifeblood. The bread represents our flesh.

We take a loaf of bread and break it in two and feed it to each other saying, "This is symbolic of my body and I'm now putting it in you." Then we serve each other wine and say, "This is symbolic of my life blood which is now your blood."

And now, symbolically, I'm in you and you're in me. We are now one together with a new nature.

Step 9—Plant a Memorial

We now leave a memorial to the covenant. We want to always remember it. We do this by planting a tree that we have sprinkled with the blood of the animal. The blood sprinkled tree, along with our scar, will always be a testimony to our covenant.

So, this completes the ceremony. From now on, we are known as friends. In Bible times, one didn't use the word friend loosely as we do today. You became friends only after you had cut covenant. And all our children are included in this covenant, even the unborn ones. They are in covenant because they are in us. Later, when they are born and come to an age of understanding about our covenant, they can choose to stay in it, or reject it.

This covenant is something special. In Hebrews 6:13 Paul states that God could find no one greater, so He cut the covenant with Himself. The explanation is found in Genesis 15:17-18, "And it came to pass, when the sun went down and it was dark, that behold, there appeared a smoking oven and a burning torch that passed between those pieces. On the same day the LORD made a covenant with Abram."

Notice that there were two beings that passed through the pieces. The smoking oven would be the Father God, the God of all Glory. The burning torch would be Jesus, the Son of God. Jesus is the fire from His loins down and from His loins up in the book of Revelation. There was no one greater, so the Father and the Son walked between those pieces of animal on behalf of Abram. Do you comprehend the significance?

If Abram had cut the covenant with God on his own, it would have been marred from God's perspective. Abram being a man, sinful by nature could easily break the covenant. God wasn't setting up a temporal covenant. It was eternal, to be replaced by the New Covenant in Christ. Abram moved aside and watched through a hazy cloud, God the Father and God the Son pass through those pieces of animal, stopping after walking their figure eight, they vocalized their promise to each other on behalf of Abram.

Imagine the wonder of Abram's heart as this impression was forever branded upon his conscience. Did you know that the impact of the New Covenant far exceeds the impact of the Old Covenant? To the natural mind you may think you have never had an experience like Abram's. However, when you met Jesus as Savior, the Glory of heaven shown in your heart without a haze. The brightness of His Glory resides in you. Paul said that we are children of light. Jesus said that you should let your light so shine before men.

Continuing on from verse 13, God revealed to Abram again the land he inherits and it's borders and also, the promise of his son to be born. This time the promise is in blood.

God's Appointed Time for the Miraculous

The next verse says that *through faith* and patience Abraham received the promise. We will have to revert back to the second chapter on expectancy to under-stand what this means. Remember, what and how you expect has to do with time. Paul wrote in Romans 4 that Abraham's faith grew stronger as he endured. How was it that with strong faith, the child wasn't born earlier?

Gen. 18:14 reads, "Is any thing too hard for the LORD? At the time appointed I will return unto thee, according to the time of life, and Sarah shall have a son." The phrase, *the appointed time*, is the key to the faith and patience needed for Abraham to have a son. The timing of Isaac to be born was in the hands of the Lord. Faith was in the hands of Abraham. Even though Abraham's faith grew stronger as he considered the promise, it couldn't make Isaac be born any faster than the appointed time.

On the other hand, if Abraham's faith had weak-ened, the appointed time would not have come. There are many things we need that may take time to believe in, however, this verse does not apply to all areas of redemption.

For example, healing has already been purchased for us. There is no need to wait for healing when in reality, it is waiting on you. If by His stripes you were healed, there is no reason for you to exercise patience with your faith. The moment you believe you receive;

healing is either instantaneously evident or it begins and you recover.

An example where patience is necessary is if God were to speak to you concerning His upcoming plans for your life. There may be a time of preparation necessary which would require the need of patience to accompany your faith.

Prosperity is a redemptive right to obtain and walk in. As the Scriptures clearly reveal, faithfully putting your hand to the plow, and sowing tithes and offerings brings prosperity. Patience is necessary because the law of sowing and reaping is part of the process. Today you sow and tomorrow there is a season of reaping.

We should never plan on waiting for any part of redemption that has already been imparted to us.

Heb. 6:16 declares, "For men indeed swear by the greater, and an oath for confirmation is for them an end of all dispute." Throughout Scripture we under-stand that the natural is explained before the spiritual so the things of God will be easily understood. Here we see the natural things men do to secure for them-selves by contract what has been agreed upon.

Men seek out those who have a greater supply for aid. Oaths and contracts are made for the fulfillment of promises. Disputes are ended when those promises are legal and binding. The law guarantees confirma-tion. The writer of Hebrews is setting us up for God's perspective on the fulfillment of a guarantee. Keep in mind that the purpose of this book is to reveal the mind of God concerning His faithfulness to fulfill His word. How bold would we be to act on the word if there was the slightest chance that God would not come through for us?

Hebrews 6:17 clearly shows us the strength of God's commitment: "Thus God, determining to show more abundantly to the heirs of promise the immutability of His counsel, confirmed it by an oath." Within the context of this chapter and book, I believe that the first two words of this verse are simply incredible: *Thus God.*

Understanding the commitments that men make with one another to legally secure promises made, can you imagine the security of having an agreement with God? Throughout the entire Bible, everything starts and finishes with God being involved. John in his gospel tells us that everything that was made was made through the Word. Nothing was made without Him. If we have an agreement where God is involved, then we have it made. Contracts, oaths, vows and promises all take on a new meaning when seen through the eyes of covenant. How awesome!

Looking at verse 17, let's go one word further. "Thus God, *determining....*" Have you noticed in the Bible there is no place where God has set out to do something where He has failed? From the beginning in Genesis chapter one, every time God said something or did something there was a creation. God saw that everything He made was very good.

Be Confident in God's Covenant Word

How does this help to establish your confidence for the future? No matter what difficulty God's people experienced, when God's purpose or determination was in action there always was deliverance and safety. It is easier to say that it would be a greater miracle if God's determined purposes were not fulfilled than if it was. It is impossible for God's purposes to fail. "For this purpose the Son of God was manifested, that He might destroy the works of the devil" (1 John 3:8). Just as God's purpose was visible through Jesus, so also, God wants His purpose visible through us.

"Thus God, determining *to show....*" Again, we see the focus of chapter three. Jehovah, the self-existing one who reveals Himself, is the God who is determined to show Himself. You would think that if God were so excited to show us His goodness that we would see more of Him in our lives. As we will see in the context of this verse, God needs our cooperation to succeed in His purpose.

Let's see what He is determined to show us. Verse 17 says that it is the immutability of His counsel. This simply means: *the unchangeableness of His purpose.* Malachi 3:6 affirms, "For I am the Lord— I do not change. That is why you are not already utterly destroyed [for my mercy endures forever]" (TLB).

In James 1:17 we read, "Every good and perfect gift is from above, coming down from the Father of the heavenly lights, who does not change like shifting shadows" (NIV). The highest revelation to man that can be obtained is through simple trust. The idea that God can be trusted to do what He said. Jesus made reference to this simple truth in Mark 10:15, "Assuredly, I say to you, whoever does not receive the kingdom of God as a little child will by no means enter it."

Consider the innocence of children; trust is simple because of total dependence. They don't have a reference point of doubt or unbelief. Total dependence causes them to believe the word of their parents without question. The world's idea of maturity is to become independent or self-reliant. Herein lies the difficulty of believing God.

We must abandon our reliance of what others say or what we know about a situation in light of what God says. The information of the world will always reveal to you what you can or cannot have, or what you can or cannot do. God's word takes the limits off your life by exploring all the possibilities of heavenly things while still living on the earth.

To live in the blessings of God demands a great maturity. Heaven's way of thinking is far beyond ours. Maturity in God is becoming fully dependent on God. Isn't this why Jesus said that the Kingdom of God must be entered with the faith of a child? It's not based on your effort, but His. What God is establishing here is man's total dependence upon the integrity of His word. Unless man responds to God in faith, God is unable to bless and provide for man. The greatest blessing God could give us would not be God making everything happen irregardless of us. God's blessing comes by giving to man the ability to trust Him, thus, the reason for the blood covenant.

Covenant Guarantees Promise

Completing the verse, we read "Thus God, determining to show *more abundantly to the heirs of promise the immutability of His counsel, confirmed it by an oath*" (Heb. 6:17 *italics added*). I love how the Lord always backs up His word with action. If the promise wasn't good enough, God cut a covenant proving the validity of the promise. This is similar to Jesus talking with the Pharisees in John 10:30, "I and my Father are one." As a result, the Jews took up stones to stone Him. Jesus replied in verses 37-38, "If I do not do the works of My Father, do not believe Me; but if I do, though you do not believe Me, believe the works, that you may know and believe that the Father is in Me, and I in Him."

God's works, not just His words, prove His faithfulness. Basically, Jesus is saying, *If you don't like the words that I speak, at least view the works and see that what I say and what I do are the same thing.* God is so interested in reaching your heart of faith, that He will demonstrate and confirm His Word just to prove Himself trustworthy. Hebrews 6:17 declares, "God also bound himself with an oath, so that those he promised to help would be perfectly sure and never need to wonder whether he might change his plans" (TLB). Keep in mind that all that is being said is for the benefit of Abram. God answered his questions thus settling forever that Abram can trust God.

God's covenant legally guarantees His promise. All that was promised Abram, God confirmed or legally settled with an oath—the cutting of covenant. This unbreakable contract is God's way of securing man's unswerving confidence. God is placing His own existence and legitimacy on the line with this oath. There would be a greater chance of birds swimming and fish flying than for God to alter this covenant.

The most unthinkable would sooner happen than for God to fail to fulfill His promise. Hebrews 6:18 confirms, "That by two immutable things, in which it is impossible for God to lie, we might have strong consolation, who have fled for refuge to lay hold of the hope set before us." God's integrity has been poured into the promise and the oath, sealing forever its truthfulness.

God never lies. Since it is impossible for God to lie, then it becomes impossible for what God has promised and what God has performed to fail. Moses reminds us in Numbers 23:19 that, "God is not a man, that he should lie; neither the son of man, that he should repent: hath he said, and shall he not do it? Or hath he spoken, and shall he not make it good?"(KJV).

Jesus emphatically underscores His Father's intentions saying in Matthew 5:18, "I tell you the truth, until heaven and earth disappear, not the smallest letter, not the least stroke of a pen, will by any means disappear from the Law until everything is accomplished" (NIV).

Covenant Security and Consolation

God in covenant has placed Himself in a position of absoluteness that gives us refuge. In covenant, we find ourselves in Christ safely and securely seated in heavenly places—the secret place. "He who dwells in the secret place of the Most High shall abide under the shadow of the Almighty. I will say of the LORD, 'He is my refuge and my fortress; My God, in Him I will trust'" (Ps. 91:1-2).

When everything seems contrary to what God has promised, His covenant oath provides strong consolation. This has nothing to do with religious piety—emotional distress that fails to deliver the necessary solution. God's strong consolation strengthens the soul, enabling it to withstand the attack of the adversary irrespective of how bad things look in the natural.

When you have nowhere to turn, no refuge to confide in, the God with whom you are in covenant will console and strengthen your soul. Paul writes in Romans 4 that with all the circumstances looking hopeless, Abraham believed in hope. When the natural gave Abraham no evidence for hope, the promise of God, unbreakable through covenant, provided expectancy for the miraculous.

Ask yourself these critical questions about covenant:

- Is it possible when the furnace is being heated seven times hotter as with the three Hebrew children, that there is a possession of expectancy for God's intervention that could calm the soul?
- Could there be a basis for definite action that would secure the blessings of God even when everything is contrary?
- When the storm is raging and the ship looks as if it is going under, what is it that strengthens the soul, and releases the power of God to calm the storm?
- What if through my mind thoughts are firing faster than machine gun bullets to enforce my utter defeat, what then am I left to believe?
- As things move from bad to worse, can I still maintain and even progress in courage to not go under, or walk through the fire and always triumph?

You can expect the miraculous in the worst of circumstances when you have a promise from God, backed by an oath. A promise and an oath is what...

- walked through the fire,
- came out of the lions den,
- took the head of a giant,

- killed 1000 Philistines with a jaw bone of a donkey,
- walked to the other side of the Red Sea on dry ground,
- raised the dead,
- opened the blinded eye,
- cleansed the leper,
- and went to a cross,
- died and arose on the third day triumphant over death, hell and the grave!

It is this hope (Heb. 6:19) we have as an anchor of the soul. If there is one thing that must be satisfied in man, it is the soul. Reason has been crowned king of the heart since the day Adam and Eve sinned in the garden. Reason is the devil's chaotic system that runs the world.

But faith, not reason, gives us ultimate hope and victory. The Apostle John wrote in his epistle that our faith is the victory that overcomes this world's system (1 John 5:4). Faith in what? Faith in God's promise and the oath it confirms.

As long as the soul roams unchecked with uncertainties, reason will dominate and control your destiny. If the devil can hold you captive to the realm of reason, he will defeat you. However, if you make him submit to the realm of faith, you will defeat him every time.

The blood covenant is the one supreme act and promise of God which has the power to quiet and even anchor the soul of man. When every natural man or woman would respond to life's trials and woes without hope, in search of man's best solution, the man or woman of God will find solitude and ultimate victory in God alone.

With your mind, will, emotions and intellect submitted and surrendered to God's Spirit through covenant, reason has no basis for complaint. As the covenant that God established is understood, your soul will come to rest and valiant actions are sure to follow.

Not a man or woman who is listed in the hall of faith found in Hebrews chapter 11 ever acted boldly without their minds being firmly established in the promises and oath of God. When this covenant was complete, Abraham never questioned God again. To Abraham, every thing God would and could say was more powerful than the world itself. Even with a seemingly contradictory request, when God required Abraham to sacrifice Isaac on the altar, he never wavered or questioned God at all.

In Hebrews 11, Abraham believed that God would raise Isaac from the ashes. The promise of God is that Isaac will be the seed through which the nations of the world will be blessed. Abraham's thoughts might have been, "And God now requires me to kill him, then the only solution can be that after I kill him, honoring the word of my covenant partner, my partner must raise him from the ashes to fulfill the original promise and oath. There is no need to worry, we are in covenant."

Our Covenant Hope is Anchored in Jesus Christ

Before we conclude this all-important teaching, isn't it interesting that the covenant with Abraham is being explained with a comparison to the New Testament covenant with Jesus Christ? The hope of our covenant is anchored because Jesus as High Priest is the one who enters in behind the veil to secure an eternal redemption forever. If Abraham's covenant so settled his conscience with only the shedding of the blood of bulls and goats, what strength of soul would come to the heart of the believer who has been washed in the blood of our Lord Jesus Christ?

We have a better covenant with Jesus, thus *the miraculous guaranteed!* We have absolutely no right to ever question the integrity of God's word. Wherever you find God's covenant promise in the Bible, God has to perform it...*if you will believe it.*

As long as the blood of Jesus is forever at the mercy seat of the heavenly altar, this covenant will never fail. The bolder you are to believe it, the better it works. Make no bones about it; this covenant is the most rock solid force in the world. Even if the heavens and earth were to pass away, the Word of God would remain. The covenant is not based on human frailties.

The Father cut this covenant with the Son hanging on the cross. The Bible is the great promise that Jesus secured for us, written in His blood. When He arose from the grave, triumphant over death and hell, He presented His blood as the eternal seal and sacrifice for man. Not the devil or one demon or all of hell put together can stop the believer who acts boldly on the covenant of the ages. Nothing could be more absolute in the entire world as God's power to back up His word.

The Bible isn't just a promise, it's a manifestation of everything that God loves about you and that God has done for you. This isn't just about what God believes about you, it's what God will do for you. Remember, God is a bottom line God. The Bible is God's action toward man.

When I started to work at the Healing School for Kenneth Hagin Ministries, I had very little experience for myself. I preached the best sermons that I could find. Within the first four months I saw many people die who believed the best that they knew how. I did the best I could, but it wasn't good enough. My sermons lacked what was necessary to deliver the power of God and stir up their faith, as it should be. Most of the messages were putting the healing off into the future. There was more emphasis placed on people recovering in time, than what God was anxiously desiring to do now.

Of course, we were teaching the people to release their faith that they had received healing, yet no one was expecting change to be right now. We sent people away believing they received, which is good, however, no one experienced their healing right then.

I don't think that Jesus would have had crowds of people following Him if He conducted His meetings that way, do you? As I began to see the power of

God's covenant to produce results, immediately I began to preach that you could expect God to do something right now. During the first week of this teaching, many wonderful miracles began to happen. Right under the palm of my hand, a growth disappeared. People were jumping up healed without even being touched.

Before that week was over the head usher said to me, "I have seen more happen this week than in all the last six years put together." When I questioned him about what he just said, he said, "I can count on one hand, how many times I've seen people healed in the last six years." Of course, we know that people were healed as they went. However, not much at all was happening in the services. This began what has been the aspiration of my life; to contend for the ministry of Jesus as He gave it to the body of Christ.

We interpret things for ourselves and have many things handed down to us through the centuries, yet whenever teaching fails to produce as the ministry of Jesus did it must be infiltrated with some type of religion. The power of God's covenant is your foundation for believing that God will do what He said He would do. In other words, He'll back you up.

Keys to Living in the Miraculous

- Live in confident expectation of miracles.

- Let your confident hope in the God of covenant prompt your faith to act.

- Walk in the covenant God has cut with you through Christ.

- Let faith in God, not reason, bring strong consolation to your soul when you are tempted to worry or doubt His promises.

- Be bold in declaring and acting by faith on God's covenant promises.

- Stand on the authority and power of God's covenant to see and do the miraculous *now!*

Chapter 5

JEHOVAH'S NAMES GUARANTEE THE MIRACULOUS!

I HAD AN INTERESTING EXPERIENCE ONE day as I was praying. I had been talking to the Lord about the need to understand more concerning His healing power. To be honest, I was feeling less than excited about what I knew and had accomplished in light of so many people who needed help. I asked the Lord a simple question which I didn't expect an answer for, 'Lord, what am I going to say today, what am I going to do?"

As if the Lord spoke audibly, I heard Him say, "Whatever you do, I'll back you up."

I had to ask the Lord to repeat that two more times so I could get it. The more I began to think about what the Lord spoke to me, the more I realized He really wanted to work with me as much as I desired to work with Him. Actually, He really wanted to be seen and known more than I was giving Him credit for.

Jesus made a comment to the Jews in John 5:20 that expresses His view of the Father's heart to reveal Himself, "For the Father loves the Son, and shows Him all things that He Himself does: and He will show Him greater works than these, that you may marvel."

Jesus was not only completely dependent upon the Father; He also constantly expected revelation to be given Him.

Jesus was expressing the character of God: that God would continually reveal Himself to us, as a benefit to us individually and for the overall purpose of fulfilling His will on the earth.

The covenant God made with Abraham didn't start and stop with the promise of a son. It was the beginning of a relationship with man that would bring progressive revelation. God used the strength of the covenant; it's ability to establish a relationship and convince man of God's reliability, to introduce His continued provision for every need of man.

As we have already seen in chapter three, once God was finished with the creation process, He immediately introduced Himself to all living things. He used the name, *Jehovah Elohim* to describe for us the way He revealed Himself. All creation understood that God was the one and only true God. Jehovah not only helps us to see God's intent to show Himself or manifest Himself to creation, but it also helps us to see the commitment involved. Jehovah is used as an everlasting covenant.

Since God revealed Himself as the one and only true God in the beginning, then you will continue to find this revelation throughout the Bible. When all is revealed in the end, everything living will acknowledge that there is one and only one true God. It's interesting to note that there was no other revelation given at this point to describe the ability or provision of God.

As Man Had Needs, God Revealed Himself

Simply put, there was no need for God to reveal Himself any other way because there were no needs. Remember that everything was already provided on the earth when man was made. Not one living thing that God created needed anything else. Sounds too good to be true, doesn't it?

This is the brilliance of the plan of God through Jesus Christ. The last Adam brought restoration to man for the areas of lack that sin produced. As good as the Garden of Eden sounds, all that provision has been reestablished. The year of Jubilee is the restora-tion of all things lost or stolen.

The premise for what shall be revealed in this chapter is the simple understanding of the Lord's Atonement. The Day of Atonement was the timetable in the Old Testament where every man would return to recover his possessions. The year of Jubilee has a divine order established in the Old Testament and completed in the New Testament. First there is the atonement, the covering of sin. Then the trumpet is sounded indicating that every one is to return to his possessions. In Hebrews we read that there is a better covenant with better promises.

With Jesus being the surety of the covenant, our sins are not covered up, they are forever remitted. As far as the east is from the west (Ps. 103:12), the sin problem has been solved through the death, burial and resurrection of the Lord Jesus Christ. If the sin problem has been solved, then all the problems birthed through sin are also solved.

The trumpet sounding in the New Testament is the heralding of the Gospel message. This message is not for the Jew alone, it's for whosoever. God recon-ciled the whole world through Christ. The very last thing that Jesus mentioned as He preached His mes-sage in the synagogues, everywhere He went, was that the anointing He was anointed with was to preach the *acceptable year of the Lord.*

This phrase is synonymous with the Year of Jubilee. This is the believer's message that everything necessary for life and godliness has been returned. Everything spiritually necessary to resurrect the will of God for your life has already been given to every believer.

Further revelation concerning God's character and ability is not seen until after man sinned and fell short of God's Glory. As man began to function within the scope of his responsibilities,

God would reveal the instructions and information necessary. Once decay set in, with the devastation of sin, man would begin to experience need.

Now suddenly, areas of man's existence that might have been taken for granted, such as the areas of need in the earth today, he would have to learn how to overcome. Through God's continued progressive revelation, man learns in what ways he can trust God and by faith receive provision.

God would not reveal anything for information alone. Everything revealed was for the express purpose of benefiting man in his need. Always remember that God is the ultimate revealer. Made in His image, we also have the responsibility of revealing God. This was the assignment of Jesus in the earth. To reveal His Father God in everything He did. Everything you learn in the Scriptures should reveal God in an area of your life.

God's Guarantee in His Names

As pointed out by Dr. Scofield concerning the Redemptive names of God, "Each one points to a continuous and increasing self-revelation." He also comments as saying, "In His redemptive relation to man, Jehovah has seven compound names which reveal Him as meeting every need of man for his lost state to the end." A look at these seven names will impart to your heart an understanding of God's great provision for you. God is definitely more than enough for every need and desires that all receive the fullness of His provision.

1. Jehovah Shammah. The most important of the seven redemptive names in my opinion is Jehovah Shammah, "The Lord is there, or present". The reason why I think that this name is so important is because every bold action of faith exists in the revelation that God is with you. When you search the Word of God, you will find that anyone who had a thorough understanding of God's abiding presence performed mighty daring feats of faith.

When God created the heavens and the earth and all living things, He did so for man. When He created man, He did so for companionship. God made man in His god class of being so He could fellowship with Him. Even the psalmist picked up on the love of God for man in Psalm 8:4, "What is man, that thou art mindful of him? and the son of man, that thou visitest him?" (KJV).

Sin is the very thing that causes man to relinquish his rights and privileges to the fellowship that he was created for. In Genesis 3:8, after man sinned, God came in the cool of the day to fellowship with Adam. The first thing that God said to Adam is, "Where are you Adam?"

Do you think that God didn't know where Adam was? Of course not, He was simply saying, "Why are you over there, when you should be over here?" Out of perfect love, God had to remove Adam and Eve out of the Garden of Eden. When He did the scriptures say that God drove Adam out of the Garden. The word "drove" means, "to apply force that cannot be withstood."

In other words, Adam did not want to go out of the Garden. Everything in him wanted to stay in that safe haven of security where he knew the comfort of God's presence. Yet it was sin and the effect of sin that made that impossible. Sin separated Adam from the presence of God on the earth. Once man exited the Garden the process of decay that sin produced in the conscience of man began its work until today. Humanity finds it very difficult to conceive of and recognize the presence of God.

What has indeed replaced the awareness of God, being theistic, is the acknowledgement of things, being materialistic. The moment man sinned, the spirit of man was dethroned and the soul of man stepped up to rule the heart of man. The will, emotions and intellect are now governed by reason.

Every person understands the war between the flesh or senses and the heart or spirit of man. Paul said in Galatians 5 that these are so contrary to one another that at times it is difficult to know what you are doing. The further the devil has exalted reason, based on the senses of the flesh, the more difficult the pathway to God becomes for man to find. Within the heart there dwells the desire to experience the purpose for existence. The ignorance of God and man's place or relationship in God has diverted man's quest to the natural realm for satisfaction. This explains why someone can climb the corporate ladder of success and still be so miserable even to the point of becoming suicidal.

Without God, everything that the world offers fails to satisfy the yearning of the human heart for purpose and fulfillment. Only Jesus can satisfy the longing in your soul. Only the reconciliation of the man on the inside, the spirit of man, can cause fulfillment to emerge. John records the purpose of man fulfilled in Revelation 3:20 where Jesus said, "Look! I have been standing at the door, and I am constantly knocking. If anyone hears me calling him and opens the door, I will come in and fellowship with him and he with me" (TLB).

I trust that those who have taken time to read this book personally know Jesus Christ as Savior. If you do not, this would be a wonderful time to call upon the name of the Lord, confessing Jesus as Lord and Savior of your life. If you do know Jesus as Lord, then your experience of receiving Him as Lord is just the beginning of a relationship that will last for eternity.

Don't wait. Enjoy the fellowship and communion of God in your soul right now. Experience the awareness and presence of God in your life today. Don't have a religion and yet deny the power or reality of God. He is there to walk with you, talk with you and share His heart with you always. You're never alone!

Throughout the Old Testament men and women who withstood the challenges of impossible odds did so because they were aware of God. Anyone who was called into ministry or hand picked on assignment was comforted with the phrase, "I will be with you."

The very thing that left the conscience of man after the fall is the awareness of God, the very thing that God instills in the soul of anyone who steps into the miraculous realm of God.

God told Moses, *Certainly I will be with you.* He told Joshua, *Be bold, be strong, for the Lord thy God is with you where ever you go.* Gideon, David, the three Hebrew children, and Daniel all were consciously aware of God.

After Elijah went into heaven in the chariot of fire, his mantle that represented God's presence, anointing and power fell to the ground for Elisha to pick up. However, what good is an animal skin if God isn't in it? The first thing that Elisha did was to test the validity of God's presence. He picked up the mantle, went over to the Jordan River and smote the waters with it while saying, "Where is the God of Elijah?"

When the waters parted as they did for Elijah, Elisha was satisfied and confident that God would do for him as he did for Elijah. Even the sons of the prophets who witnessed this miracle said, "The spirit of Elijah now rests on Elisha."

Let me insert here a new creation reality. Under the Old Testament not every one was anointed with the presence of God. Only the Prophet, Priest and King and sometimes a called out judge of the Lord were anointed. Everyone else lacked the personal touch of God. When the children of Israel were to meet God at the Mountain of Horeb, God gave spe-cific instructions to the children of Israel not to touch Mt. Sinai.

In the New Testament this personal touch of God on man is made available for everyone who receives it. There is no need to question whether or not God is with you. Why, because the great mystery of the church that Paul was given was, "Christ in you, the hope of glory" (Col. 1:27).

God comes personally to live inside each child of God. We become the temple of God, the home where God lives. We don't need to strike the water to see if God is there. Instead, we strike the water *because He is there*. Running, dancing and shouting would be appropriate at this point!

A fascinating verse of scripture that continues to reiterate the need for us to be reminded that God is *Jehovah Shammah*, the God who reveals His presence, is found in the book of Acts. Acts 10:38 says, "How God anointed Jesus of Nazareth with the Holy Ghost and with power: who went about doing good, and healing all that were oppressed of the devil; for God was with him" (KJV).

Look at the last five words of this statement concerning Jesus' ministry, "...for God was with him." My book, *Until I Come*, stressed the importance of adopting the mentality of Jesus in order to do the works as He did. If you study the ministry of Jesus throughout the Gospel of John, you will find that Jesus continually talked about His relationship and confidence with the Father.

If the confidence and comfort of knowing that "God is with us" was important to Jesus, how much more so should it be to us. Jesus became so use to the companionship of the Father, that while hanging on the cross, He cried out when the Father left Him. When sin separated Jesus from His Father, He cried out, "My God, My God, Why hast thou forsaken me?"

Jesus became as we were, so that we could become as He is. Drawn into union, we have been made one with Jesus. Maybe having experienced it for himself, Jesus knew that the disciples would need reinforce-ment and encouragement when He was gone. Before He left, Jesus said, "Lo, I am with you always, even unto the end of the age." John records Jesus preparing His disciples for the day when He would leave as say-ing in John 14:16-20, "And I will pray the Father, and he shall give you another Comforter, that he may abide with you forever; Even the Spirit of truth; whom the world cannot receive, because it seeth him not, neither knoweth him: but ye know him; for he dwelleth with you, and shall be in you. I will not leave you comfortless: I will come to you. Yet a little while, and the world seeth me no more; but ye see me: because I live, ye shall live also. At that day ye shall know that I am in my Father, and ye in me, and I in you" (KJV).

Notice that Jesus went one step further than the idea that the Holy Spirit would be with the disciples. He said that the Holy Spirit would also live in them. It was this presence of the Holy Ghost that fell on the Day of Pentecost and radically changed the perspec-tive of the disciples so much so that confidence in the endowment of power made them irresistible to the world.

Miracles are commonplace to the person who knows God. Would David have run towards Goliath without God being there? Is it possible that you haven't been running towards your giant because you're wondering what will happen if what you believe in doesn't work?

Believer, take heart! God is in covenant with you for the very purpose of revealing His presence always. John 14:21 declares, "He that hath my commandments, and keepeth them, he it is that loveth me: and he that loveth me shall be loved of my Father, and I will love him, and will manifest myself to him" (KJV). *Jehovah Shammah* is God's covenant of Glory, the manifest presence of who He is.

2. **Jehovah Rapha.** I'm sure you can see the significance of starting with *Jehovah Shammah*. If God is truly with us, then all that He is is with us at all times. It's much easier to understand these things from the other side of the cross. During the Old Testament, men were experiencing God step by step. Let's look at the covenant name for healing in the physical body. *Jehovah Rapha* is translated, "I am the Lord thy Physician" or "I the Lord make you immune to sickness" or "I am the Lord that healeth thee."

When the children of Israel passed through the Red Sea they came to the waters of Marah that were bitter and unhealthy. God showed Moses a tree, from which Moses threw part of it into the water to cure the bitterness. God established an ordinance there saying, "If you diligently heed the voice of the LORD your God and do what is right in His sight, give ear to His commandments and keep all His statutes, I will put none of the diseases on you which I have brought on the Egyptians. For I am the LORD who heals you" (Exodus 15:26).

To understand this through the eyes of the atonement, you would need to see Jesus fulfill this revelation in the New Testament. As you would imagine, the ministry of Jesus was not complete without great numbers of healings taking place.

Note this interesting truth. God healed the waters at Marah before He ever revealed the knowledge that He could always be counted on as the Lord, our great Physician. Do you see that God is more willing to get the waters healed for the benefit of the people, than He is to announce to everyone that He is something special? The revelation of who God is, is only to perpetuate an ever-lasting covenant for divine health.

Isaiah wrote about this redemptive work in Isaiah 53:4-5, "Surely he hath borne our griefs, and carried our sorrows: yet we did esteem him stricken, smitten of God, and afflicted. But he was wounded for our transgressions, he was bruised for our iniquities: the chastisement of our peace was upon him; and with his stripes we are healed" (KJV).

Jesus is the fulfillment of this scripture, which prophesies the redemptive work of the Lord.

Remember, for God to reveal a redemptive name in the Old Testament, there must be a fulfillment in the New Testament. Matthew 8:16-17 declares, "When the even was come, they brought unto him many that were possessed with devils: and he cast out the spirits with his word, and healed all that were sick: That it might be fulfilled which was spoken by Esaias the prophet, saying, Himself took our infirmities, and bare our sicknesses." (KJV).

It should be quite clear that this covenant that God made with Moses in Exodus 15 is fulfilled satisfactorily through the ministry of Jesus. Jesus not only walked on the earth as the fulfillment, but He successfully arose triumphant over all the work of sickness and disease to forever prove His role as Healer of all sickness and disease. The great emphasis of this covenant is the actual work of deliverance performed on the human body to keep one free from all sickness and disease.

Are you living in the joy and reassurance that God, *Jehovah Rapha*, has made a covenant proving to you His desire and faithfulness to show up in your body as healer and caretaker of your temple, the body in which God dwells? (1 Cor. 3:16, 6:19) Your body is the temple of the Holy Ghost, the place where He dwells.

There is no corruption in God's house in heaven, so God has seen fit to provide through His covenant an ample supply of health and healing for the rest of your time on this earth. The Lord is truly our healer, our life support and the one who makes us immune to all sickness and diseases.

While Jesus walked on the earth, multitudes followed after Him to receive His teachings and the benefit of healing to their physical bodies. When Jesus would come to a town, people would recognize Him and bring all the sick folks to get healed. The question I want to ask is, "What happened if you were two or three towns away from Jesus and you needed a healing now?"

If you couldn't get to him and he couldn't get to you, you would die. This is where the song, *Cum By Ya* gets sung. Come by here, come by here, you can sing this until the cows come home and you won't get healed unless Jesus comes. Thank God for redemption. Once and for all, Jesus comes to live in you, taking up residence. You'll never have to sing, come by here. *Jehovah Rapha* has already come; everything you need for health and healing is already yours!

3. **Jehovah Jireh.** This name of God means, "Jehovah sees." It's the symbolic name revealed to Abraham on Mount Moriah in commemoration of the interposition of the Angel of Jehovah (Yahweh) who prevented the sacrifice of Isaac and provided a substitute offering to God.

Abraham used this name to identify God's provision at the altar of sacrifice. In Genesis 22:13-14, we read, "And Abraham lifted up his eyes, and looked, and behold behind him a ram caught in a thicket by his horns: and Abraham went and took the ram, and offered him up for a burnt offering in the stead of his son. And Abraham called the name of that place Jehovah-jireh: as it is said to this day, In the mount of the LORD it shall be seen" (KJV).

In Genesis 22, God asked Abraham to take his son and sacrifice him on an altar. This was the son of covenant whom God said would be the beginning of many descendants that would out number the stars in the sky. Now God was asking Abraham to sacrifice Isaac.

I want you to see how important it was that there was a ram caught in the bush. Being the *great provider*, God is also the *great planner*. He sees ahead of your need, and makes provision before you think you need it. God didn't just zap a ram into the bush for Abraham at the exact moment. That ram was already singled out for the assignment that Abraham's faith would fulfill.

In the light of the name Jehovah, *the self existent one who reveals Himself*, God desires that you experience His provision. In John 5, Jesus talked about seeing the work of His Father and making provision. "Jesus replied, 'The Son can do nothing by himself. He does only what he sees the Father doing, and in the same way. For the Father loves the Son, and tells him everything he is doing; and the Son will do far more awesome miracles than this man's healing'" (John 5:19-20 TLB).

The ability to see the provision before the need is something Jesus relied upon for His faith in demonstrations. Jesus said in Matthew 6:8, "Therefore do not be like them. For your Father knows the things you have need of before you ask Him" (NKJ).

The application of this understanding made Jesus immoveable when confronted with need. His knowledge of God's supply produced expectancy for the needed provision. In John 6, Jesus was faced with the hunger of a multitude. In verse 5 Jesus asked Phillip, "Where shall we buy bread, that these may eat?"

Then John wrote in verse 6, "But this He said to test him, for He Himself knew what He would do." God is your great provider. *Jehovah Jireh is* the one who sees the need before the need and makes abundant provision before you need it most.

4. **Jehovah Shalom** is the name for, the Lord is our Peace. "And the angel of God said unto him, Take the flesh and the unleavened cakes, and lay them upon this rock, and pour out the broth. And he did so. Then the angel of the LORD put forth the end of the staff that was in his hand, and touched the flesh and the unleavened cakes; and there rose up fire out of the rock, and consumed the flesh and the unleavened cakes. Then the angel of the LORD departed out of his sight. And when Gideon perceived that he was an angel of the LORD, Gideon said, Alas, O Lord GOD! For because I have seen an angel of the LORD face to face. And the LORD said unto him, Peace be unto thee; fear not: thou shalt not die. Then Gideon built an altar there unto the LORD, and called it Jehovah-shalom: unto this day it is yet in Ophrah of the Abi-ezrites" (Judges 6:20-24).

In the sixth chapter of Judges God visited Gideon to raise him up as a deliverer to the people of Israel. Because of Gideon's hesitancy to except the position, God worked with Gideon to convince him of God's loyalty to defeat the Midianites. As we pick up with the progress of the Lord in verses 20-24, God is performing one of Gideon's last requests to convince him of His faithfulness.

Notice in verse 21 that once the angel of the Lord departed Gideon finally understood what was happening. He realized that his experience was indeed a visitation of the Lord. When fear struck his heart, God removed it with peace. Peace is the solution to every turmoil or storm in life. Isaiah informs us that in the atonement Jesus took the chastisement of our peace upon Him.

All the punishment that man deserved was laid on Jesus. When Jesus proclaims that His peace is what He gives us, and this peace is not as the world gives, our hearts should cease to be afraid. There is no need for concern or worry since Jesus has carried the stress of every impossible situation; conquered the stress and overcame the impossible.

Jesus was straightforward in informing us that in this world there would be trials and persecutions (John 16:33). However, He encouraged our hearts by overcoming every one of them. Truly Jesus is our peace, our wholeness and freedom from all chastisement.

5. **Jehovah Nissi** is the name for; the Lord is our banner, victor or captain.

> *Then came Amalek, and fought with Israel in Rephidim. And Moses said unto Joshua, Choose us out men, and go out, fight with*

> Amalek: tomorrow I will stand on the top of the hill with the rod of God in mine hand. So Joshua did as Moses had said to him, and fought with Amalek: and Moses, Aaron, and Hur went up to the top of the hill.
> And it came to pass, when Moses held up his hand, that Israel prevailed: and when he let down his hand, Amalek prevailed. But Moses' hands were heavy; and they took a stone, and put it under him, and he sat thereon; and Aaron and Hur stayed up his hands, the one on the one side, and the other on the other side; and his hands were steady until the going down of the sun. And Joshua discomfited Amalek and his people with the edge of the sword.
> And the LORD said unto Moses, Write this for a memorial in a book, and rehearse it in the ears of Joshua: for I will utterly put out the remembrance of Amalek from under heaven. And Moses built an altar, and called the name of it Jehovah-nissi. (Exodus 17:8-15 KJV)

Jehovah Nissi represents God's covenant with Abraham in whom He states that He is a Shield and exceedingly great reward. Simply put, the Lord will fight for us. Many times through out the Old Testament, the phrase, "stand ye still and see the salvation of the Lord" was given in the midst of battle. God's position has always been to defend His own. In Exodus we can see the significance of Moses holding up the staff, which represents the presence of God. God fighting for us doesn't mean there is nothing for us to do. As we stand our ground in faith, there is no weapon formed against us that shall prosper (Isa. 54:17).

Through the atonement of the Lord Jesus Christ we see the ultimate banner of our salvation. Colossians 2:15 reads, "Having disarmed principalities and powers, He made a public spectacle of them, triumphing over them in it." *Phillips* translation reads, "And them, having drawn the sting of all the powers ranged against us, He exposed them, shattered, empty and defeated, in His final glorious triumphant act." Also, the *Cotton Patch* translation says, "And having frisked the top brass and the power boys, and made them prisoners of war, He publicly exposed them."

Jesus is the Captain of our Salvation, the banner that goes before us as the King of kings and the Lord of lords. What is this ultimate victory without our experience of it? It's dry religion, denying the power of His resurrection. Remember, He is *Jehovah Nissi*, the one who reveals or manifests complete victory. Thank God we always triumph through our Lord Jesus Christ.

6. **Jehovah Ra'ah** translated is "The Lord is my Shepherd."

> *For thus saith the Lord GOD; Behold, I, even I, will both search my sheep, and seek them*

out. *As a shepherd seeketh out his flock in the day that he is among his sheep that are scattered; so will I seek out my sheep, and will deliver them out of all places where they have been scattered in the cloudy and dark day. And I will bring them out from the people, and gather them from the countries, and will bring them to their own land, and feed them upon the mountains of Israel by the rivers, and in all the inhabited places of the country.*

I will feed them in a good pasture, and upon the high mountains of Israel shall their fold be: there shall they lie in a good fold, and in a fat pasture shall they feed upon the mountains of Israel. I will feed my flock, and I will cause them to lie down, saith the Lord GOD. I will seek that which was lost, and bring again that which was driven away, and will bind up that which was broken, and will strengthen that which was sick: but I will destroy the fat and the strong; I will feed them with judgment. (Ezek. 34:11-16 KJV)

The atonement is the giving of one life for another. *Jehovah Ra'ah* is the one who reveals himself as the great substitute. Jesus proved this through redemption. In John 10:11, Jesus said about Himself, "I am the good shepherd: the good shepherd giveth his life for the sheep." Of course, the greatest summary of Jesus as the shepherd is given in Psalm 23 which begins, "The LORD is my shepherd; I shall not want."

As our Shepherd, the covenant-making God, *Jehovah Ra'ah*, has promised to guide, direct, comfort and care for us in every situation. We have nothing to fear, not even death itself, with God shepherding us.

7. **Jehovah Tsidkenu** is the covenant name for, "The Lord our Righteousness." We read in Jeremiah 23:5-6, "Behold, the days come, saith the LORD, that I will raise unto David a righteous Branch, and a King shall reign and prosper, and shall execute judgment and justice in the earth. In his days Judah shall be saved, and Israel shall dwell safely: and this is his name whereby he shall be called, THE LORD OUR RIGHTEOUSNESS."

One of the most needed truths to convince the world of is still that Jesus became our righteousness as He bore our sins on the cross. The gift of righteousness is God's gift to you regardless of what you have or have not done. There is no merit outside of the legal justification of Christ. God declares you righteous on account of the work Jesus did. This eliminates the unworthiness and condemnation that hinders the majority of believers from receiving. Righteousness is God's qualification for your every need and provision.

To completely understand the importance of this teaching on God's covenant names, which guarantee the miraculous in our lives, I want you to see what

Paul prayed in Ephesians through the Amplified version of the Bible. Ephesians 3:18-19 declares, "...that you may have the power and be strong to apprehend and grasp with all the saints (God's devoted people, **the experience of that love**) what is the breadth and length and height and depth of it; that you may really come to know—**practically, through experience for yourselves**—the love of Christ, which far surpasses mere knowledge **(without experience);** that you may be filled through all your being unto all the fullness of God—that is, may have the richest measure of the divine Presence, and become a body wholly filled and flooded with God Himself!"

Do you understand the importance Paul places on the experience of God? For too long we have tried to direct people's experiences to line up with the word, so that we have almost eliminated the experience altogether. We have become accustomed to attending meetings where the Word is preached with no demonstrations, and believing that everything is okay. Granted, I know that there are different kinds of services and that each has its own purpose.

However, Jesus rarely targeted an area of doctrine without the people receiving results. This is what made Jesus' ministry so different from the Pharisees. They had only a form of doctrine, but there was no liberating power to set people free.

The covenant was ordained for the purpose of producing an expectancy in our daily lives for miraculous results. Why would God's people ever be nervous in any life-threatening situation, if they were in covenant with a God who would bring the experiences of their covenant into reality.

If the covenant wasn't any good, then you wouldn't have good experiences. However, if the covenant provided protection and care for all of man's needs while on the earth, you could then expect to experience all of the goodness of God.

God's constant presence, divine health, complete provision, undeniable peace, victorious protection, loving care, restored well-being and confidence in life are available to all who believe. That includes you. Believe it...God's covenant names guarantee the miraculous in your life now! Believe it today!

Keys for Living in the Miraculous

- Believe that God has revealed Himself in His names to keep His covenant promises to you.

- **Today** *Jehovah Shammah* is present with you in every circumstance of life.

- **Today** *Jehovah Rapha* is your health and your healing.

- **Today** *Jehovah Jireh* will provide for all your needs.

- **Today** *Jehovah Shalom* brings a calming peace to every storm of life.

- **Today** *Jehovah Nissi* is the banner over you declaring victory.

- **Today** *Jehovah Ra'ah* shepherds you through every valley.

- **Today** *Jehovah Tsedkenu* clothes you in the righteousness of His Son Jesus Christ, and redeems you from every sin.

- Declare the names of God in every situation knowing that His promises are sealed and guaranteed by His Name

Chapter 6

GOD'S MIRACULOUS WAYS

For of Him and through Him and to Him are all things. For all things originate with Him; all things live through Him, and all things center in and tend to consummate and to end in Him. To Him be Glory forever! Amen, so be it" (Romans 11:36, AMP). What a glorious prayer!

In every age, humanity has been thoroughly awe struck over the miraculous and mysterious ways of God. We have heard the religious try to explain natural catastrophes by saying, "God's ways are mysterious you know." In one sense, the realm of God or the unseen world will always be mysterious. Will we always think of God as the one who giveth and who taketh away? Should we always be in the dark as to the operations of God and our expectancy for them?

If faith is the heart response that releases the

promises of God, then how could we be so unaware of the method God uses to fulfill our faith? For faith to be backed with substance or power, we need to know with certainty what can be expected from God. On the other hand, if prayers continue to exhibit the uncertainty of this religious plea, "If it be thy will," then faith cannot be used effectively. We must know how God does what He does, so we can cooperate with Him efficiently and pray effective prayers (James 5).

God Reveals the Ways He Works

Psalms 103:7 opens up the possibilities of faith on a whole new level, "He made known His ways to Moses, his acts to the children of Israel." The difference between Moses and the children of Israel is understood by what they knew. They both saw the works of God in their completed form.

God took Moses one step further though, he was blessed to know *how God did what He did*. The ben-efit is obvious. Moses learned how to work with God on the level where God produced results. Moses then became a viable tool on the earth for the sake of con-tinually manufacturing results.

Let me explain this to you with an analogy. If I can go behind closed doors and find out how something is done, then I not only have the privilege of using the finished product, but I am now instrumental in the production of the product. Doing the works of Jesus on the earth has so much to do with understanding how God accomplishes what He does.

Paul wrote in Colossians 1:9, "Be assured that from the first day we heard of you, we haven't stopped praying for you, asking God to give you wise minds and spirits attuned to his will, and so acquire a thorough understanding of the ways in which God works" (The Message Bible). God wants us to have a thorough understanding of the ways in which He works.

Can you imagine being an employee trying to do a good job, yet your employer never communicates well the assignment? How difficult is it to give your all, knowing that it might be all wrong? A lack of confidence always shows up in the way things turn out. Giving someone the greatest opportunity to achieve good results begins with good communication. Proper instructions and guidelines create a healthy environment for success. Would God commission us to do the works of Jesus and not adequately communicate our assignment? Of course not!

"For of Him and through Him and to Him are all things..." (Rom. 11:36). This verse reveals that there is an organized beginning and ending to all things. I usually draw a circle to examine this verse. The circle represents a completed project, or a manifestation of God's Word. There is rhythm and divine reason to every manifestation in God. Our investigation is based on the finished work of Christ. Jesus understood how to work within the framework of how God does what He does.

In John 9:3-4, Jesus revealed the heart of God concerning the will of the Father. He said concerning the blind man, the works of God should be manifest in him. Then Jesus revealed that there is a method to working with God. He said in verse 4, "I must work the works of God." Jesus recognized the part He had in the overall working of God to accomplish the will of God.

Going to the book of beginnings, Genesis, will help us locate God and His methods of operation. Genesis 1:1 reveals, "In the beginning God created the heavens and the earth." Let's establish a rule: *whenever we see the name God within the context of what He is doing, this name represents: God the Father, God the Son and God the Holy Ghost.* All three are involved here with creation. As we develop this thought further, you will see that God does not create independent of each other as separate personalities. Everything revealed in this natural world is done by the Trinity.

God Originates or Initiates All That Is

Reading Romans 11:36, the verse begins with, "For *of Him*...." A scripture that explains this divine personality is 1 Corinthians 8:5-6, "Yet for us there is one God, the Father, *of whom* are all things, and we for Him; and one Lord Jesus Christ, through whom are all things, and through whom we live."

Notice that in the phrase, *of whom*, the *whom* is speaking about the Father. If we use our circle as an illustration, the Father would be at the top. "Of whom are all things," is a phrase depicting the Father as the originator of all things. This means that God the Father is the architect who designs the blue print for whatever is created. Is this the reason why Jesus was so insistent on following the will of the Father?

In John 6:38 Jesus said, "I came not to do my own will, but the will of my Father who sent me." It's not as though the only person who can think is the Father. Everyone has the capacity to reason and arrive at conclusions for their life. It's just that the Father's position as the originator of all thought gives Him superiority in this area.

Psalms 37:23 says, "The steps of a good man are ordered by the LORD, And He delights in his way." You can choose your own path. However, the path of the Lord is best. Jesus did have a human will. We see Jesus struggling between two wills in the garden of Gethsemane. Jesus prayed, "Let this cup pass from me, not my will, but your will be done." As the son of Man, Jesus' will wrestles momentarily with the ultimate decision in front of Him—going to the cross. Though tempted as we are, Jesus *always* makes the right decision. He submits His will to the Father. The Son *always* acts as the Father wills.

Jesus knew and we must never forget that God is the originator of all that is. He is the master designer, the omniscient mind of God that knows always the highest and best.

So let's return to our illustration of the circle. At the top of the circle is God the Father, the Creator, who originates all things. As we move around the circle which represents moving from God's will to God's action, we come to the Son who incarnates God's will. That is to say, that the Word or Will of God becomes flesh, i.e. takes on human form in words and actions which perfectly live out in time and space the invisible, perfect will of God.

So what begins as invisible, for God is a Spirit, and what He wills is revealed first in heaven. That invisible will becomes visible as the Son speaks and acts upon the will of the Father. Interestingly, the Hebrew word for "word" is *davar*. *Davar* means both to act and to speak. The Hebrew word for truth is *amet*, which denotes absolute consistency between what is said and what is done. Jesus is both the Word (*davar*) of God (read John 1) and the Truth (*amet*) of God (read John 14). So when Jesus speaks or acts, He does with absolute consistency exactly what the Father wills.

Once the Son speaks and acts, the Holy Spirit manifests or produces the good work or fruit of the work of the Father so that the invisible becomes visible (read 2 Cor. 4:17-18) and that good work and fruit glorifies the Father. So, going back to our circle, we have moved from God the Father and Creator on the top of the circle, around to the bottom of the circle with Jesus the Word speaking and acting upon God's will, now proceed back to the Father by the Holy Spirit. The Spirit thus manifests or produces the good fruit and good works that return glory to the Father. Thus the full circuit is completed and the

Trinity has been involved in all things as Romans 11:36 has revealed.

Let's use another word picture. If the structure that we're investigating could be demonstrated on the earth, it would resemble a corporation. God the Father would then be the CEO of the corporation. The plan, the design and the strategy would evolve from Him. In any corporation there is more working to produce an outcome than just the head. There must be those who are able to implement the plan.

Jesus Speaks and Acts Out the Will of God

The second part of implementation is the Son. 1Corinthians 8:5-6 says, "...and one Lord Jesus Christ, through whom are all things, and through whom we live." Romans 11:36 shows us that the second part of the Trinity is the "through Him" personality. In the corporate setting, who is the "through him" person? It's the middle manager—that person responsible for consulting with and having the mind of the CEO. Jesus consults with and has the mind of the Father.

The responsibility, however, doesn't end with middle management. Now you must adequately communicate direction and inspiration to those who must implement the plans and produce the results. The effectiveness of communication from the CEO through the manager to the helpers or workers will greatly affect the outcome. I believe we could call this position the helpers or the workers. Now then, the

Holy Spirit whom Scripture calls the Helper refers to the fruit of what is *manifested* as "the work of the Holy Spirit."

A point worth noting is that all things are of the Father and all things are through the Son. This means that both the Father and the Son each share equal responsibility to produce all things. As we examine the ministry of Jesus, we find Jesus speaking the invisible into the visible as He teaches us to pray "...Your kingdom come, Your will be done on earth as it is in heaven" (Matt. 6:10). Jesus was interested in revealing the will of God on the earth. He had an unusual job showing and declaring to people the Father when no one can see Him.

Even in a corporate structure, if the CEO is not visible, then it is the responsibility of the manager to produce results so every one can see the CEO through the product produced. In John 10:30 Jesus said, "My Father and I are one." The Jews took up stones to stone Him. Jesus answered by saying, "For which of these good works do you stone me?" Jesus used the works produced to validate His relationship with the Father.

In John 14:8-11 Philip said, "Lord, show us the Father and that will be enough for us." Jesus answered, "Don't you know me, Philip, even after I have been among you such a long time? Anyone who has seen me has seen the Father. How can you say, 'Show us the Father'? Don't you believe that I am in the Father, and that the Father is in me? The words I say to you are not just my own. Rather, it is the

Father, living in me, who is doing his work. Believe me when I say that I am in the Father and the Father is in me; or at least believe on the evidence of the miracles themselves" (NIV).

Jesus' position was crucial concerning the outcome of anything that God wanted established on the earth. He managed to bring the invisible to the visible so that His followers could implement the will of the Father through the power of the Holy Spirit.

John 1 sheds further importance to the ministry of Jesus on the earth. "In the beginning was the Word, and the Word was with God, and the Word was God. He was in the beginning with God. All things were made through Him, and without Him nothing was made that was made" (John 1:1-3). Without Jesus, nothing was made that was made. We could safely say that because we are the body of Christ, then nothing in our lives will be completed without Jesus being involved. "He [Jesus] is the image of the invisible God, the firstborn over all creation. For by Him all things were created that are in heaven and that are on earth, visible and invisible, whether thrones or dominions or principalities or powers. All things were created through Him and for Him. And He is before all things, and in Him all things consist. And He is the head of the body, the church, who is the beginning, the firstborn from the dead, that in all things He may have the preeminence" (Col. 1:15-18).

Notice that in Jesus "all things consist." In other words, in Christ all things are held together. Nothing has substance without Him. Could it be that if all the heavenly blessings have already been given to us that within the plan of redemption all things pertaining to the well-being of our lives consists within Christ? If this were true, then it would make sense to understand how Jesus worked within the structure of the corporation of God.

When Jesus walked on the earth, He did so as a human being. All of His knowledge was learned. He developed His earth walk in the time He spent with heavenly things. The real secret to Jesus' life can be seen in John 3:13, "No one has ascended to heaven but He who came down from heaven, that is, the Son of Man who is in heaven." As you can see, it looks as if Jesus is in two places at the same time. He was in contact with heaven and earth simultaneously.

As a human being, we are in contact with two worlds at the same time. Our body is necessary for the operations of this world and our spirit is necessary for the spirit world. If we were to choose which world has greater potential, then it would be the spirit world. It was the spirit world that created this natural world. Things unseen created the things that are seen.

Because we, as human beings, represent a link between the two worlds, then we can choose which realm to represent. Jesus was God's expression of a human being submitted to heaven's will. The word "submission" is a key word in Jesus' ministry and life. Without His consecration to the will and purpose of His Father, He would have been living only to establish His own will. But being fully committed to God's will, Jesus managed to bring heaven to earth and fully submit, as a human being, to the divine will of God.

All that is necessary to live in the miraculous as Jesus did, is to follow God's ways. Remember that Jesus gave us the advantage of the Holy Ghost to do so. We can be committed to God's ways as Jesus was. What did His commitment look like? Two scriptures show us the commitment of Jesus:

> *Therefore Jesus answered and was saying to them, "Truly, truly, I say to you, the Son can do nothing of Himself, unless it is something He sees the Father doing; for whatever the Father does, these things the Son also does in like manner. For the Father loves the Son, and shows Him all things that He Himself is doing; and the Father will show Him greater works than these, so that you will marvel."* (John 5:19-20 NASU)
>
> *"For I did not speak on My own initiative, but the Father Himself who sent Me has given Me a commandment as to what to say and what to speak. I know that His commandment is eternal life; therefore the things I speak, I speak just as the Father has told Me."* (John 12:49-50 NASU)

There are two ways for a human being to express themselves. They are through 1) words and 2) actions. The main reason why the writing of this material is so important for us is that we need our minds renewed into the mind of Christ. The mind definitely influences the expressions of a human being. Jesus became so knowledgeable and committed to the will of the Father that His expressions were perfectly executed. If we'll remember that there are three personalities, then we'll come back to the worker's or helper's position in manifesting what the Father willed and the Son speaks and acts upon.

The Holy Spirit Helps to Manifest Fruit

Romans 11:36 reads, "For of Him and through Him and to Him are all things, to whom be glory forever, Amen." After revealing the positions of the Father as the originator of all things and Jesus the Son as the One who speaks and acts upon holding all things together, there is only one personality left for "to Him." God the Holy Spirit is the "to Him," the finisher of the circle.

In the beginning when God created, it was all three divine personalities involved. Each had His own responsibility, yet all equal in their importance. Without each one being involved, there would be no creative work. In the ministry of Jesus, He waited until the endowment of power was upon Him to begin His public ministry. The endowment of power was the Holy Ghost. Luke 3:21-22 declares, "Now when all the people were baptized, it came to pass, that Jesus also being baptized, and praying, the heaven was opened, And the Holy Ghost descended in a bodily shape like a dove upon him, and a voice came from heaven, which said, Thou art my beloved Son; in thee I am well pleased" (KJV).

The Holy Ghost must have something to do with the finished result. Paul writing to the Corinthians concerning spiritual things calls the Holy Ghost, the One who manifests. 1 Corinthians 12:7 "Now to each one the *manifestation* of the Spirit is given for the common good" (NIV).

The word manifestation means "to show, to exhibit or to uncover." The Holy Ghost or Holy Spirit is the one who provides the manifestation. The "to Him" personality is the one who finishes the plan that was originated in the heart of the Father and that was spoken and acted upon by the Son.

In Mark 16 we are given the great commission by our Lord as the responsibility of the church to complete the will of God on the earth. Mark 16:15-20 reads:

> *And then he [Jesus] told them, "You are to go into all the world and preach the Good News to everyone, everywhere. Those who believe and are baptized will be saved. But those who refuse to believe will be condemned. And those who believe shall use my authority to cast out demons, and they shall speak new languages. They will be able even to handle snakes with safety, and if they drink anything poisonous, it won't hurt them; and they will be able to place their hands on the sick and heal them."*

> *When the Lord Jesus had finished talking with them, he was taken up into heaven and sat down at God's right hand. And the disciples went everywhere preaching, and the Lord was with them and confirmed what they said by the miracles that followed their messages.* (TLB)

As the disciples were instructed, they were to preach the gospel message. As we can see, when the message was preached, the Lord would be present to confirm the message. The word, "confirm," means to remove doubt by an authoritative act or indisputable fact.

In the gospel of John chapters 14 through 16, Jesus spent a considerable amount of time convincing the disciples that in His absence they would have another Helper. The Holy Spirit would be sent in place of Jesus to carry on the work of Jesus. So when we see the Lord present to confirm the message, the scripture is talking about the Spirit of the Lord or the Holy Spirit.

So, the Holy Spirit would work with the Word to produce indisputable facts. Confirmation is the finishing touch to the Word of God. How important is confirmation to the Word? It is the validation of whether or not the Word is true. Isaiah 55:8-11 declares how important it is to God that His word be confirmed, "This plan of mine is not what you would work out, neither are my thoughts the same as yours! For just as the heavens are higher than the earth, so are my ways higher than yours, and my thoughts than yours. As the rain and snow come down from heaven and stay upon the ground to water the earth, and cause the grain to grow and to produce seed for the farmer and bread for the hungry, so also is my Word. I send it out, and it always produces fruit. It shall accomplish all I want it to and prosper everywhere I send it" (TLB).

Verse 11 tells us what happens when the word is acted on, it always produces fruit. In John 15:8, Jesus tells us that the Father is glorified by much fruit. Glorified means a work of glory or the sum total of God's manifestations has been accomplished, the outcome is much fruit.

Jesus waited to begin His public ministry until He was baptized in the river Jordan. At that time, the Holy Spirit like a dove came upon Him. Remember, the presence of the Holy Spirit is the finishing touch. Jesus' first miracle was in Cana, where He turned the water into wine. John 2:11 reads, "This beginning of signs Jesus did in Cana of Galilee, and manifested His glory; and His disciples believed in Him."

The Holy Spirit is the manifesto, the Glory of the Father. His work always produces fruit. Fruit produced glorifies the Father because His word accomplished what it was intended to do. The Holy Spirit's position is vital to the confirmation of the Word of God. When Jesus told the disciples to wait in the city of Jerusalem to be endowed with power from on high, He was talking about the baptism of the Holy Spirit.

Having traveled with Jesus for three years, Peter was aware of how to use the power of the Holy Spirit. Speaking to the man at the entrance of the temple, Peter commanded him to rise up well in the name of Jesus. The man was made whole. This is fruit. It couldn't have happened without the presence of the Holy Spirit. This is why Jesus told the disciples to tarry in the city of Jerusalem until they received the power of the Holy Spirit (read Acts 1).

Later the disciples were questioned by the Pharisees about the miracle that took place with the crippled man. Peter said that faith in the name of Jesus made the man whole. The Pharisees were indignant and wanted to eliminate Peter and John. The sole reason why they couldn't is because the people beheld a notable miracle. That was confirmation!

The Holy Spirit Confirms God's Will for the Miraculous

The apostle Paul was a stickler for the word having confirmation. He used to be a zealous Pharisee, completely adhering to the law. His understanding of the law was a compiling of rules and regulations. There was no Spirit involved. Once Paul was converted and filled with the Holy Spirit, Jesus explained to him the importance of the power of the gospel.

Paul writes in 1 Corinthians 2 his method of operation as he preaches the gospel. "When I came to you, brothers, I did not come with eloquence or superior wisdom as I proclaimed to you the testimony about God. For I resolved to know nothing while I was with you except Jesus Christ and him crucified. I came to you in weakness and fear, and with much trembling. My message and my preaching were not with wise and persuasive words, but with a demonstration of the Spirit's power, so that your faith might not rest on men's wisdom, but on God's power" (1 Cor. 2:1-5 NIV).

Paul was set on not delivering the Word of God without the demonstration of the Spirit's power. The word demonstration means, "to manifest, to show off, or to exhibit." Paul expected the word preached to be met with the showings off of the Holy Ghost. The Word preached will make room for an exhibition of the power of God. The further we explain the function of the Holy Ghost, the greater will be your expectation of His working of the miraculous.

In Paul's letter to the Roman believers, Paul explained that while we were still sinners Christ died for us. This Paul called love in demonstration. God is all about action. You couldn't in any way classify God as we might talk about a dog that is all bark but no bite. God says what He means, and means what He says. If He says He is *Jehovah Rapha*, the God that heals, then you can count on a demonstration of healing.

In a corporation the CEO needs individuals to deliver the vision and watch over it to ensure its completion. The completion is accomplished by individuals who actually do the assembly of the product.

Their responsibility is to follow the instructions of the manager by accurately creating the vision of the CEO. Thus the cycle is complete. The limitations of poor communication and human failure are eliminated in the Godhead. God runs a perfect corporation without failure, and on time deliveries.

As the Body of Christ, we must pay close attention to the actions of Jesus. Now that the three divine personalities are defined, the whole corporation begins to make sense. We have already seen how important the plan of the Father is to Jesus. He stayed completely committed to the words and actions of the Father. If the Holy Ghost is also submitted to the plan of the Father, then you can see the importance of Jesus adhering with specifics to the plan.

In Matthew 5:18 Jesus said, "I tell you the truth, until heaven and earth disappear, not the smallest letter, not the least stroke of a pen, will by any means disappear from the Law until everything is accomplished" (NIV). When Jesus described the Holy Spirit, He called Him the Spirit of Truth. It would be impossible for the Holy Spirit to manifest anything except the truth. This certainly puts pressure on us to know and act on the word. Jesus not only relied on the words and actions of the Father, but He also fulfilled the written word.

In Matthew 8:16-17, "When evening had come, they brought to Him many who were demon-possessed. And He cast out the spirits with a word, and healed all who were sick, that it might be fulfilled which was spoken by Isaiah the prophet, saying: 'He Himself took our infirmities and bore our sicknesses.'" As long as Jesus brought the word to the trials of life, He was confident of the Holy Spirit being involved.

John wrote about confidence in 1 John 5:14-15, "This is the confidence we have in approaching God: that if we ask anything according to his will, he hears us. And if we know that he hears us-whatever we ask- we know that we have what we asked of him" (NIV). When the Word is involved, we have absolute confidence that we have the desired result. In other words, when the Holy Ghost is in operation, we have results that manifest the will of God. As I look at Jesus, I can see His trust in the plan of the Father, and complete confidence in the Holy Spirit.

Be Confident in the Father, Son and Holy Spirit

There is an important point that must be understood if optimal confidence is to be exercised. Going back to the creation process, we find an interesting function of the Holy Spirit which should eliminate all fear of failure when believing God. Genesis 1:1-2 reads, "In the beginning God created the heavens and the earth. The earth was without form, and void; and darkness was on the face of the deep. And the Spirit of God was hovering over the face of the waters." As we mentioned earlier, when we see the name God here, we are referring to the divine Trinity. My question would be, "Who was the first divine personality of the Divine Trinity mentioned in the Bible?"

The answer would be found in the second verse, "the Spirit of God." Maybe as a result of divine order we would have thought that the Father would be mentioned first. Or from the beginning, the emphasis should have been on Jesus. Yet as you can see, God's order and method of operation puts the Holy Spirit's place as the first mentioned.

My statements concerning this subject are with great respect to the Father of whom are all things. I'm very aware that for the Holy Spirit to be mentioned first as an individual personality, it must mean that the Father had already originated the plan. Everything begins in Him.

Why would the person of the Holy Spirit be mentioned first? I believe that God is setting a precedent in the beginning of the Bible that will be established throughout the scriptures. A revelation to the church that once received in the heart would forever empower us to act courageously in faith.

If God is extremely willing to manifest His truth to our hearts and lives, then the messages He writes in His word should inspire us to act in faith. Before we conclude the reason why the Holy Spirit is mentioned first, let's see what He was doing as He was mentioned. Verse two says, "...And the Spirit of God was hovering over the face of the waters." Look at the verb, *hovering*. The word **hover** means to brood, to hatch or incubate.

As Webster's Dictionary points out, to **incubate** means, to sit on eggs so as to hatch by the warmth of the body. The word **incubation** means:

1. Process of incubation.
2. The period between the infection of an individual by a pathogen and the manifestation of the disease it causes.

The word **incubator** means an apparatus with a chamber used to provide controlled environmental conditions especially for cultivation. As you can see, the Spirit of God was warming things up for the Word to be spoken. If we will remember the progres-sion of the Godhead, we know that the Holy Ghost always responds to the Word in action.

However, isn't it interesting to see His foreknowl-edge concerning the mind of God, and then the activity He engages in before His turn is called on? Let's look at a sports team to see if these principles hold up. On a football team the coach calls in the play for the quarterback to run. The play must be executed correctly in order to have success.

The quarterback calls the play and then takes his position to run the play. The whole team now knows the mind of the coach. They all visualize their assign-ments and prepare to fulfill them. Let's say, the play is a pass to the wide receiver. That receiver has to go to a place and occupy it before there is a completion of the pass. What would happen if the receiver falls down, and the quarterback throws the pass with an expectation that the receiver would be there? The pass is incomplete.

However, if the receiver runs His route well, then he will be where he needs to be when the ball comes. If he waits for the ball to be thrown, before he runs to his spot, it may be too late. Jeremiah 1:12 says that God "hastens to perform His word." 2 Peter 3:9 in Weymouth's translation reads, "God is not slow in fulfilling His promise, He bears patiently, waiting on you."

If God is waiting on us, then He must be in the right place, the place of your manifestation before you need Him. This is why the Holy Ghost was hovering over the face of the waters before the words "Let there be light" were spoken. The Holy Ghost was there ahead of time, preparing the environment so that the *manifestation* of the will of God acted on would be timely.

Paul said in Philippians 2:13 (Amplified) that, "it is God who is all the while at work in you, creating and empowering you with desire and ability to do of His good will, satisfaction and delight." If the eyes of the Lord are roaming throughout the entire earth, isn't it because He is seeking to demonstrate His love? Or is God a giant egomaniac who thrives on attention? How about this, God loves us so much that He is moved continually by His heart of compassion to be on display for our well-being and benefit.

The Holy Spirit is that person of the Godhead who will bring the desired result when we act on the Word.

If the action of the Word always brings the function of the Holy Ghost into play, then this describes the reason why Jesus was so confident as the living Word of God. Jesus in His earthly walk was the divine expression of God. He was the Word in action.

How could you fail if the Word is always supported with the power of the Holy Spirit? God the Father did not release His plan with failure built into it. God is not a man that He should or would lie. Remembering the fourth chapter in this book, God set up the covenant on purpose to establish the authenticity of the Word of God. Whatever has been spoken by God must come to pass.

Throughout the gospels we see Jesus continually manifesting power as it were, at will. However, as you have seen, this isn't hocus-pocus. There is a method to the manifestation of the Spirit. If you think back to Moses at the Red Sea, this is why God told Moses to raise the rod and split the sea. Without Moses doing the Word, the Holy Spirit would have been inactive in producing the manifestations of power. God had already told Moses that the signet of His power was in the rod.

Moses had to think like God and act like Jesus which would reveal the power of God, the Holy Spirit. We, in turn, are to think like God and act like Jesus if we are going to see any change on the earth. God backing you up is as simple as your willingness to act and continue to act on the Word.

If the Holy Spirit's position is preceded by His preparation of the environment where the Word will be acted on, then you have nothing to fear. He's not just there on time, He's ahead of time. Could this make us bold like Jesus, speaking and stepping out with confidence in the Father's word or will and total trust in the Holy Spirit to perform?

The purpose of this book is to convince you of God's willingness to be where you need Him to be so His Word will be revealed in your life. Just as God showed Moses His ways, God will show you His ways!

Living in the Miraculous

- Trust God the Father to initiate and originate every plan for good in your life.

- Like Jesus did, manage, speak and act upon God's will for your life.

- Trust the Holy Spirit to manifest good fruit in your life to glorify God.

- Begin to act upon God's Word knowing that the Spirit has already incubated a miracle to be manifested as you boldly, without fear, trust the Holy Spirit to perform and produce the miraculous!

Chapter 7

PRACTICING THE REALITY OF THE MIRACULOUS

Jesus declares, "But he that doeth truth cometh to the light that his deeds may be made manifest, that they are wrought in God" (John 3:21 KJV). For the body of Christ to rise to the level of the early church and beyond, there must come to the hearts of its members the boldness and confidence that Jesus portrayed throughout His earthly ministry.

After seeing how the Godhead cooperates with one another, we are ready to more thoroughly discuss the position of the initiator. Jesus' emphasis here in John 3:21 is on being a "doer of truth." James in his letter wrote that *hearing the word without being a doer of the word is to deceive oneself* (James 1:21). God's purpose in giving us the Word is to establish correct thoughts. God the Father has given us His thoughts written in the Word of God to provide the information of our covenant rights.

The power of the Word is that it is empowered by the Holy Ghost. The inspiration of God is breathed into the Word, making it come alive in your heart as you hear it. If the Holy Spirit inspired men as they wrote it, then the inherent ability of God continues to reside within the Word to inspire you as you read it. Also, if the Holy Spirit moved upon the Holy men of old to write the scriptures, then the Word with its ability to inspire you will move you to act on it as you read it.

The principles may be the same as one being inspired to act on something learned naturally. However, there is a great difference, namely God. When God gets involved there is always change. We are never changed in the presence of men or circumstances but we are always changed in His presence by His Word and through His Spirit.

John 3:20 begins with, "for everyone practicing evil." The word *practice* is used in verse 20 and the word *doer* is used in verse 21. I would like to use a synonym for "doer" which is the word *practicing* in verse 21, which would read, "for everyone practicing the truth...."

Practice Spiritual Things!

The word *practice* helps me to understand that in order to walk with God, you must develop in the spirit. Continuing to practice means that we are becoming proficient in the things of God. We can become experts in the realm of the Spirit. To watch the lives of some, you would think that maybe they have an advantage in spiritual things. Maybe their special experience qualifies them to believe God better than you.

The real truth is that everyone has the same capacity for greatness in God as the next person. The more spiritually in tune you become the easier it will be to work with God. Remember this: as born-again spiritual beings we have a greater aptitude to experience the fullness of God than our natural man has to breathe air.

I realize that you have been breathing air involuntarily while you read this book, however, you are not a physical being, you are a spiritual being. The physical is only the outerwear to the man on the inside. Peter called your spirit man the hidden man of the heart. If you are a spirit, then spiritual things ought to be the easiest things you do.

I want you to be confident that as you practice spiritual things, you will become proficient at them.

John records that we are to practice the truth. In the Greek, the word for truth means *reality*. The greatest place to start when discovering reality is, "In the beginning, God...." In others words, before we begin anything we must start with God. God's very presence births or creates everything.

We ask ourselves, "What is reality?" We must start with the beginning of all things—God. Even Jesus said the same thing in John chapter 14, "I am the way, the truth and the life." John also records what Jesus said in John 17, "Sanctify them by thy truth, thy word is truth." Two absolutes that we know to be truth: one is God and the other is God's Word. When we think of practicing reality, we must consider practicing what God has said.

We live in contact with two worlds at the same time. While most naturally we know that our bodies contact this physical world, our spirits at the same time contact the spirit world. To deny the spirit world is to forsake the power that can change this natural world. All throughout the Bible a common thread is seen: *those who utilize the help and assistance of God always win*. It's just that simple, reality is God, and everything else is very secondary.

Paul helps us understand reality with a very interesting paradox. The *Message Bible* says in 2 Corinthians 4:18, "There's far more here than meets the eye. The things we see now are here today, gone tomorrow. But the things we can't see now will last forever." What does Paul mean by there's far more here than meets the eye. The NKJV says, "While we do not look at the things which are seen, but at the things which are not seen. For the things which are seen are temporary, but the things which are not seen are eternal."

Notice the words, *things* and *seen*. Each of these words is in each phrase. So there are things that are seen and things that are not seen. We could say that the things that are not seen are just as real to the spirit realm as the things that are seen in the visible realm, that realm discerned by the senses.

Ever said about a spiritual truth, "That simply doesn't make *sense* to me"? The truth is that many spiritual truths in Scripture cannot be discerned or perceived by our natural senses. God says in Isaiah 43:19, "See, I am doing a new thing! Now it springs up; do you not perceive it?" (NIV). God's new thing is always birthed in the invisible. *Seeing* for us is never first in the natural or the visible. It's in the super-natural or the invisible.

Seeing Spiritual Reality

Our perception of reality must be transformed by the Spirit. In the past, we only saw with our natural eyes and perceived reality through our natural senses— vision, hearing, touching, tasting and smelling. But now, being born again or born of the Spirit, we can *see* or perceive things spiritually. So Paul writes in 1 Corinthians 2:11-12, "For what man knows the things of a man except the spirit of the man which is in him? Even so no one knows the things of God except the Spirit of God. Now we have received, not the spirit of the world, but the Spirit who is from God, that we might know the things that have been freely given to us by God."

Jesus made a comment to Nicodemus in John 3:12, "I have spoken to you of earthly things and you do not believe; how then will you believe if I speak of heavenly things?" (NIV) When we begin to discuss the involvement of two worlds at the same time, it becomes very important that we're able to separate the reality of both worlds. Unless this is done, it will be too easy to revert to what is familiar.

The natural world has always been so vivid to our senses. It is a process to familiarize us with new surroundings. Even naturally, it takes approximately six weeks to form a new habit. Think of Jesus in His surrounding. Every one was so aware of the natural. Jesus was all alone in the midst of unbelief. He maintained His place in God by constantly talking about heavenly things and by staying in perfect fellowship with the Father.

To clearly understand what the two worlds look like as they merge together, we'll look at 2 Kings 6:8-17:

> *Now the king of Syria was making war against Israel; and he consulted with his servants, saying, "My camp will be in such and such a place." And the man of God sent to the king of Israel, saying, "Beware that you do not pass this place, for the Syrians are coming down there." Then the king of Israel sent someone to the place of which the man of God had told him. Thus he warned him, and he was watchful there, not just once or twice.*
>
> *Therefore the heart of the king of Syria was greatly troubled by this thing; and he called his servants and said to them, "Will*

> you not show me which of us is for the king of Israel?"
> And one of his servants said, "None, my lord, O king; but Elisha, the prophet who is in Israel, tells the king of Israel the words that you speak in your bedroom."
> So he said, "Go and see where he is, that I may send and get him."
> And it was told him, saying, "Surely he is in Dothan."
> Therefore he sent horses and chariots and a great army there, and they came by night and surrounded the city. And when the servant of the man of God arose early and went out, there was an army, surrounding the city with horses and chariots. And his servant said to him, "Alas, my master! What shall we do?"
> So he answered, "Do not fear, for those who are with us are more than those who are with them." And Elisha prayed, and said, "LORD, I pray, open his eyes that he may see." Then the LORD opened the eyes of the young man, and he saw. And behold, the mountain was full of horses and chariots of fire all around Elisha.

As this story unfolds, we see two armies entangled in possible war. Through God's intervention, Israel is continually saved from Syrian attacks. To the Syrian King, it's as though someone is a traitor, selling out the Syrian army. When the King learns that it's a prophet for Israel that hears the words of the King in his bedchambers and relates them to the King of Israel, he inquires of his whereabouts. After learning he can be found in Dothan, he sends an army to capture him. They surround the city at night. This, in itself, illustrates the point that we're making, there are two worlds working at the same time.

The understanding of the spirit world will always give an advantage. As you would imagine, surrounding the city at night wouldn't take Elisha by surprise. He has already proven that with God's help the knowledge of the whereabouts of the enemy king isn't a problem. Although correct military strategy has been issued by King Ahab, it doesn't make sense when you factor in God.

In the morning, Elisha's servant went outside their tent. To his amazement there was an army fully armed and in position to capture Elisha. If you were responding from what your eyes were beholding, you would be terrified. He went back into the tent and said to his master, "What shall we do?" He only saw the natural. His perception of reality was limited to his natural senses. But Elisha could see the spirit world as well.

What about yourself? Have you been saying, "What are we going to do?" If so, you can be sure that you have been looking at the natural. Why? Because we have trained the senses so well, instinctively they have the dominant voice. The possibility that there may be another option gives you a choice. Whether or not you recognize the options is the reason for this chapter.

To See the Spiritual, Abandon Fear!

Elisha's response begins our journey into the supernatural. His words to the servant were, "Do not fear." The first thing that leaves you in the midst of your trial when you consider God's ability is fear. Fear is one of the greatest deterrents to faith. Fear is simply the expectation of bad. Fear is only present when the symptoms or circumstances have been accepted as fact. For the majority, this acceptance of symptoms or circumstances is standard. In fact when a believer chooses to believe God, most people and even other believers, think that they are crazy or foolish. Isn't that amazing?

You are foolish because you trust in the most reliable solution the world has to all of life's problems. This is the low ebb that Christianity has sunk to. We have lost our standard measurement of success—namely our relationship with Jesus Christ. When you were born again you gave Jesus your heart so He could meet every need you would ever have.

Elisha continued his response by saying, "Those who are with us are more than those who are against us. To the eye of the spiritual man, there were four groups of beings present. To the servant and the army there were only two groups of people present. Yet Elisha includes two other groups of beings. Those who were with them represent the demonic spirits from Satan. Those who are with us, represent the angelic hosts from God.

To validate this let's see what the servant of the man of God saw. Elisha prayed to God to let his servant's *spiritual* eyes open up. As the man of God prayed for the servant's eyes to open, his servant saw spiritual reality.

Paul prays for the church's eyes to open. Paul spends more time praying for spiritual eyes to open, as he preaches the Word, than the desperate prayers for God to do something as we do today. As the servant's eyes were open, he beheld horses and chariots of fire surrounding the enemy and the demon spirits. What I find to be so comforting is that Elisha was completely satisfied and confident to know that God's support was greater than the natural circumstances that so outnumbered them.

Can you see that no matter how traumatic your trial or circumstances are, they are only temporary? As long as God still has a voice, nothing is impossible. You could say that if God is for you and the whole world is against you, it wouldn't matter. You would say this not because you are going under, but because the natural has no power to control the supernatural when a man or woman believes God. Can you see how insignificant the natural is when considering God's ability?

Act Upon the Truth of Spiritual Reality

We are talking about practicing reality. Practicing reality is seeing what God sees and then by faith acting upon the truth that God has revealed to our spirit man instead of fearing the circumstances sensed by our natural man.

There is no doubt that Satan uses the natural circumstances of a cursed world to persuade the believer and the unbeliever alike to accept what comes to them. John 8 has a wonderful expose' on this subject. John 8:32 reads, "And you shall know the truth, and the truth shall make you free." Jesus begins by stating that there is freedom in reality.

I think you will agree that truth or reality by itself will not set you free. It is the truth you know and then act upon that sets you free. Knowing what is real, and then acting accordingly will definitely liberate you.

Peter began to learn to see the spiritual truth as he followed Jesus. We read in Matthew 16:13-18:

> *When Jesus came into the coasts of Caesarea Philippi, he asked his disciples, saying, whom do men say that I the Son of man am?*
>
> *And they said, Some say that thou art John the Baptist: some, Elias; and others, Jeremias, or one of the prophets.*
>
> *He saith unto them, But whom say ye that I am?*

> *And Simon Peter answered and said, Thou art the Christ, the Son of the living God.*
>
> *And Jesus answered and said unto him, Blessed art thou, Simon Barjona: for flesh and blood hath not revealed it unto thee, but my Father which is in heaven.*
>
> *And I say also unto thee, That thou art Peter, and upon this rock I will build my church; and the gates of hell shall not prevail against it.* (KJV)

If Jesus, being the Christ, the Son of the living God will keep the gates of hell from prevailing against the church, then why hasn't this reality worked? The truth is that Jesus is the Christ, the Son of the living God. Although this truth rules supreme in the realm of the spirit, it must be responded to on the earth to be established here.

The spiritual truth is this: Jesus is the Christ and when that is received in the heart of a man or woman, that spiritual truth will stop the gates of hell from prevailing against you. The great redemption truth of the work of Jesus Christ is that He reconciled the whole world unto Himself when He was justified in the spirit. On the account books in Heaven, the world has had the blood of Jesus applied.

However wonderful this may sound, it still doesn't change anything within the human heart until the truth is known and then *acted upon*. At that moment, Jesus becomes the Lord of one's life and what was legal in the spiritual world now becomes manifested and reality in the visible world.

Just because the great redemption truth exists for all humanity doesn't mean the devil won't try to keep you from knowing that it exists. If the devil had to do it all over again, he never would have crucified the Lord of Glory. But since he made that mistake, he now works night and day to keep the world ignorant to the truth.

John 8:42-44 shows us the real truth concerning the devil. "Jesus said to them, 'If God were your Father, you would love Me, for I proceeded forth and came from God; nor have I come of Myself, but He sent Me. Why do you not understand My speech? Because you are not able to listen to My word. You are of your father the devil, and the desires of your father you want to do. He was a murderer from the beginning, and does not stand in the truth, because there is no truth in him. When he speaks a lie, he speaks from his own resources, for he is a liar and the father of it.'"

Jesus reveals in verse 44 that the devil does not stand in the truth, because there is no truth in him. Therefore, if you hold the devil by faith to the truth of the Word, you will defeat him every time.

Jesus continues to say that the devil is a liar. His resources are lies. His lies are in relation to the truth. Everything that the devil uses to deceive us will be contrary to what is real in God. He will twist and distort what is real to make you think you are being religious, when in fact you're being deceived.

The name Satan means deceiver. To deceive is to cause one to roam or stray from the truth. The devil's accusations are an attempt to make you accept and act on lies that will kill, steal and destroy you (John 10:10). 2 Corinthians 11:14 says, "And no wonder, for Satan himself masquerades as an angel of light" (NIV).

In other words, Satan is a master illusionist. He is good at making something appear as if it's real, but it's not. He wants so badly to replace God. Of course he never will because the best he can do for a short time is to pervert and distort things.

How important is recognizing what is true and what isn't? It's so important that either God will be working with you or you'll be going it alone. Jesus told us that the advantage that we would have in life would be the Holy Ghost. In John 14 and 16 Jesus said that the Holy Ghost is also called the Spirit of truth. As we've learned, the word *truth* means *reality*. The guide that has been sent to lead us through this valley of the shadow of death is the Spirit of reality, i.e. truth.

In every situation we can conclude that the Holy Spirit will show us what is real. Not only is the word the deciding factor of truth, the Holy Spirit continues to provide revelation and an inward witness to the believer that will not fail.

Light Reveals Truth

"But he that doeth truth cometh to the light that his deeds may be made manifest, that they are wrought in God" (John 3:21 KJV). Returning to the text at the beginning of this chapter, Jesus said, He that practices what is truth or reality comes to the light so that His deeds may be manifest.

When light is mentioned in relationship to God it always represents His power or the work of the Holy Ghost. Light is not an independent substance; it comes from a source of energy. The sun shines because of the energy or makeup of the sun. The light is only the byproduct of the sun.

Likewise, God is light because He is life. There is no darkness in Him because there is no death in Him. God is the source of life itself. John said in chapter one, that in Him was life, and the life was the light of men. Paul calls the believer a child of the light. The only way we can be considered a child of the light is to be born of the life and nature of God.

This is why eternal life is such an important new creation reality to become aware of. Jesus was different in His earth walk from any other man because He was a vessel of divine life. The light is the power of the Holy Spirit. Jesus destroyed the works of the devil with the light. Acts 10:38 declares, "...how God anointed Jesus of Nazareth with the Holy Spirit and with power, who went about doing good and healing all who were oppressed by the devil, for God was with Him."

If a work of God is going to be accomplished, it must be done in the light. Everyone wants God to work miracles in their lives, yet they persist to act on lies. If you want the anointing to stay active in your life, you will have to practice the truth. Your words and actions will have to stay based on the Word. If you say one thing and act in a contrary way you will be deceiving yourself. 1 John 1:6 reads, "If we say that we have fellowship with Him, and walk in darkness, we lie and do not practice the truth."

As you can see, your words and actions will have to stay consistent with truth if you desire to have the anointing working with you. Throughout this book, I have detailed the reasons why you can believe that God is desirous of manifesting Himself to you. The experience of this confidence comes as we act on the Word.

You may be thinking that you have heard all your life that you need to act on the Word. It may seem like an old phrase to you. The difference is that now you know and actually expect God to perform His Word *as you act on it*.

We have so cautiously tested the Word of God, now it's time to become real doers of the Word. The doer knows that as he acts upon truth, the Spirit's power will be released to him to solve the difficulty.

Now Is the Time to Get God Involved!

Discovering the reality that God is more than willing to assist us in every endeavor of life will do us little good unless we become daring and bold to confront our challenges with faith. These thoughts are to challenge you, the believer, to get God involved in every area of your life.

Get God involved in your finances. For example, in your finances, it's essential to get God involved. You can pray all you want to, but when it comes down to the truth of the matter, are you tithing and giving offerings? Is God first in your priorities concerning money? If practicing reality means anything, then if you are faithfully abiding by the laws of increase, it would be impossible to stay broke. Giving of your tithes and offerings is in obedience to the Word, ten percent on the tithe and what ever the Lord says to you concerning the offering. In the manner that you give, it will be given back to you.

The anointing will always cause increase. When Jesus obeyed the unction of the Father concerning the multiplying of the fish and the loaves, was the anointing involved? The anointing to increase followed the action of faith. Let's release the anointing to bring increase in our lives.

Get God involved in your marriage. What about our marriage or families, how will they become blessed? Certainly, it's not by complaining about everything that is wrong. The Word of God doesn't give us the right to complain and fuss about others. If we want relationships to change, wouldn't it be good to get God involved?

As much as you might want your spouse to change, are you obeying the command that God gave you concerning them? Husbands love your wives, and wives respect your husbands. The exercises that God gives us to do are not just psychologically the best things you could do in the natural to encourage harmony; they are the pattern of spiritual truths set in the heart of God in heaven that will invoke the blessing and anointing of God to bring change.

God's desire is that His will in heaven be established on the earth. If the ways of heaven are to respond in the God kind of Love, then the anointing will not work with you unless you do. It's always easier to blame others for what is not working, but truthfully, what God will do for you is not dependent on the work of others. It's up to you.

Get God involved in your parenting. Instead of only repeating to your children what your parents said to you, begin only saying to your children what the Father tells you to say. Only do to your children what the Father tells you to do. Resist any error from previous generations by letting God's truth set you free from the past and letting His Spirit empower you to do what is right. Be an example of truth for your children.

Get God involved at the workplace. Treat your colleagues at work the way God would treat them, not the way you might respond in the natural with vengeance, greed or offense. Become forgiving. Be a light in darkness. Set an example of excellence. Be a servant.

Get God involved at church. Church isn't a religious institution—it's a gathering place for believers to worship and serve God and then minister to one another and the world. Church isn't about coming to a building or a service; it's about coming to God. See the church as the spiritual reality it is—the bride of Christ.

Where do you need to get God involved right now in your life?

All of creation is waiting for the sons of God to manifest as Paul writes in Romans 8:19. So, now is the time that we, as believers, develop and mature in spiritual things until we master the affairs of life. We are supposed to know what we're doing to bring God on the scene. Go through a checklist of the problems that face you. Bring each one of them into the light of God's word.

Now, begin to meditate on God's Word until you see yourself in the light of truth. Simply respond to what is real because it is real, even if everything seems to tell you it's not so. At this point, you can be assured that the anointing is with you. Why not act like the anointing is working. Colossians 2:12 says, "... having faith in the working of God which raised Jesus from the dead." Go ahead and believe that change is manifesting.

Remember, if Elisha could be bold because the angels of God outnumbered the demonic spirits of Satan irregardless of how bad the natural looked, how much more insistent could you be, seeing that God not only is for you and with you, but that He with all His power and might lives in you. Ask yourself the question, what is reality?

Living in the Miraculous

- See the invisible with your spirit man.

- Act boldly in faith upon the truth that Christ has revealed to you.

- Abandon the paralysis of fear and step out in faith that acts.

- Only say and do what the Father tells you by His Spirit of truth to say and do.

- Get God involved in every area of your life—home, family, marriage, workplace, church and world.

- Become light in darkness so that the world around you can see the reality of God's anointing and glory manifested in your life

Chapter 8

ABIDING IN THE VINE

I wonder sometimes why we make things so difficult that God makes so easy. It's amazing how insecure we are after being brought up in a hostile world. Fear has a hold on more of us than we know. We choose to doubt God with our own interpretations of what we would like the Word of God to say to compensate for our lack of confidence.

Much of our doctrine is clouded in unbelief. There was a time when we could have stepped out boldly to believe the Word, but because the fear of failure was unconsciously embedded in us, we sidestepped what the Word said to cover up for our unbelief. Dangerous doctrine has been taught for years through the minds of men who fail to produce results themselves. Rules and regulations, which were nailed to the cross, have been taken down and inserted once again as the crutch necessary to explain away our failures. In doing so, we blame God for not being faithful.

Jesus remarked in Mark 10:13-16, "People were bringing little children to Jesus to have him touch them, but the disciples rebuked them. When Jesus saw this, he was indignant. He said to them, 'Let the little children come to me, and do not hinder them, for the kingdom of God belongs to such as these. I tell you the truth, anyone who will not receive the kingdom of God like a little child will never enter it.' And he took the children in his arms, put his hands on them and blessed them." (NIV)

To reiterate the words of Jesus, anyone who will not receive the kingdom of God like a little child will never enter it. The emphasis of this statement seems to indicate the innocence and simple trust of a child. In the natural, as children are born, they are completely dependent upon the parents for assistance. We call a child growing up into maturity, one who learns to effectively lead an independent life.

Training a child to properly make decisions and to more than adequately function in life would be a natural goal. Even though this idea could be translated to spiritual development, there is a different approach to the end result. Of course, we want to develop spiritually where we are making proper decisions that will shape and mold our tomorrows.

Learning to obey the Lord and follow Him are tremendous aspirations. Where the natural child is born fully dependent and learns to develop into independence, it's just the opposite in the spirit.

When we are born again, our spirits are made perfect, yet our thoughts are still like they used to be. In other words, we are very independent from God. Because it seems natural to make all the decisions based on the knowledge of the past subjects learned, we struggle with submitting our will to God.

As we grow spiritually, our will becomes subjected to the will of God by our minds being renewed to the Word of God. The more we respond to the will of God, the more dependent we become on God.

During the first few months at our Healing School, we failed to get consistent results. For that matter, we hardly had any results. I remember the day when I said to the Lord that I was willing to accept the responsibility for the lack of results. Instead of blaming the people, I told the Lord it was my fault. Then I said, "As of today, I consider myself to know nothing. Lord teach me. I completely lean upon you." From this point the revelation came and so did the healings.

Jesus teaches us, "I am the Real Vine and my Father is the Farmer. He cuts off every branch of me that doesn't bear grapes. And every branch that is grape bearing he prunes back so it will bear even more. You are already pruned back by the message I have spoken. 'Live in me. Make your home in me just as I do in you. In the same way that a branch can't bear grapes by itself but only by being joined to the vine, you can't bear fruit unless you are joined with me.' I am the Vine, you are the branches. When you're joined with me and I with you, the relation intimate and organic, the harvest is sure to be abundant. Separated, you can't produce a thing. Anyone who separates from me is deadwood, gathered up and thrown on the bonfire. But if you make yourselves at home with me and my words are at home in you, you can be sure that whatever you ask will be listened to and acted upon. This is how my Father shows who he is—when you produce grapes, then you mature as my disciples." (John 15:1-8 *The Message* NT)

What a wonderful real life illustration Jesus gives us to relate our relationship with Him and the Father. As a branch we receive the life of the vine as surely as we are connected to the vine. Everything necessary for the production of fruit is in the vine.

Barclay's translation of Ephesians 1:3 reads, "Praise to the God and Father of our Lord Jesus Christ, for he in the heavenly places has blessed us with every spiritual blessing, because our life is bound up with the life of Christ." Johnson's translation says, "I can only say 'praise God' for his gifts to us through Christ, who revealed both our possibilities and the power to actualize them." Notice in the Message Bible translation above, that not choosing fellowship with the vine will have consequences. "Separated, you can't produce a thing."

The very thing that glorifies the Father is the production of fruit. The more productive we become the greater our trust is revealed in Him.

The fact that we are connected to the vine is the starting point for all things in Him. Life was never abundant in the vine that it did not supply the branches with the power of creation. Even though you would naturally think the life of the vine would flow unhindered to the branches, in the Christian's experience, how receptive the individual is to the ability of God determines the amount of life experienced.

In John 15:7 Jesus says emphatically, that if you abide in me and my word abides in you, you will ask what you desire and it will be given to you. The Christian experience basically originates in two things.

1) Fellowshipping with the Word of God.
2) Communing with the Spirit of God through prayer.

God desires His children to abide with Him always. The word "abides" means "to dwell with someone on a continual basis." We could say at this point that faith will be ineffective without fellowship with the Father.

In Proverbs 4:20-23, we read:

My son, pay attention to what I say;
Listen closely to my words.
Do not let them out of your sight,
Keep them within your heart;
for they are life to those who find them
and health to a man's whole body.
Above all else, guard your heart,
for it is the wellspring of life. (NIV)

As you can see from the writings of Solomon, the importance of undivided attention is crucial to the results we so desperately seek. One of the most challenging jobs I've done was that of a substitute teacher. Your success has everything to do with making a connection with the students. If I were to walk into a classroom and the students were engaged in conversation, but not willing to listen to me, the teacher, then we are going to have problems with conveying the material.

My first step is to get their attention. Once I have it, I have to maintain it. One of the greatest tools of the enemy is to keep your focus on everything in this life but God.

A great story that illustrates the importance of the word and the spirit to produce victories in life is found in 1 Samuel. The story of David and Goliath is a real life expose depicting the believer overcoming the adversary. 1 Sam 17:1-10 reads:

> *Now the Philistines gathered their armies together to battle, and were gathered at Sochoh, which belongs to Judah; they encamped between Sochoh and Azekah, in Ephes Dammim. And Saul and the men of Israel were gathered together, and they encamped in the Valley of Elah, and drew up in battle array against the Philistines. The Philistines stood on a mountain on one side, and Israel stood on a mountain on the other side, with a valley between them.*

> *And a champion went out from the camp of the Philistines, named Goliath, from Gath, whose height was six cubits and a span. He had a bronze helmet on his head, and he was armed with a coat of mail, and the weight of the coat was five thousand shekels of bronze. And he had bronze armor on his legs and a bronze javelin between his shoulders. Now the staff of his spear was like a weaver's beam, and his iron spearhead weighed six hundred shekels; and a shield-bearer went before him. Then he stood and cried out to the armies of Israel, and said to them, "Why have you come out to line up for battle? Am I not a Philistine, and you the servants of Saul? Choose a man for yourselves, and let him come down to me. If he is able to fight with me and kill me, then we will be your servants. But if I prevail against him and kill him, then you shall be our servants and serve us." And the Philistine said, "I defy the armies of Israel this day; give me a man, that we may fight together."*

This scenario is nothing new to the Israelites. As the children of God they have been continually harassed by the adversary, in an attempt to overthrow God's people. The Israelites would always win no matter how big the opponent, if they followed God. God had proven Himself faithful over and over again.

As you follow the tactics of the enemy throughout the history of the Bible, you find that he has stayed consistent to his method of destruction. The Garden of Eden is where the first temptation to man is witnessed. The devil uses accusations that caused man to question the legitimacy of God's word and the ability of God to back it up. Reason is the number one tool the devil uses to redirect your attentions away from the simple trust of God's word. Reason is released through the senses. However, things you hear, see, feel, taste and smell in this world are not the only sources of information that exist. If your senses are tuned into the world, then everything that comes down the pike will be processed as a legitimate source of information.

The only thing that will break this cycle is a personal time of fellowship with the Word of God and God Himself. The greater awareness you have developed of God and His Word, the less likely you will fall for the temptations in the world.

In the story above, Goliath represents the devil and the armies of the Lord represent the believer. As we begin you can see that both sides are lined up against one another. Paul remarked in Gal 5:16-18, "I say then: Walk in the Spirit, and you shall not fulfill the lust of the flesh. For the flesh lusts against the Spirit, and the Spirit against the flesh; and these are contrary to one another, so that you do not do the things that you wish. But if you are led by the Spirit, you are not under the law."

You must understand that the adversary is

arrayed against you. Your senses live in a negative world that transmits ungodly signals to your brain constantly. These signals will, if unchecked by the Word of God, lead you to disobey God. It's not a good enough idea to put your brain in neutral and coast through life. If you are not purposefully maintaining a healthy thought life, an unhealthy thought life will exist. There is a working out of our salvation that will produce a spiritualization of our soul so closely knit to the will of God that our senses will be exercised to understand and discern both good and evil.

Don't Listen to the Devil!

As we read the dialogue of Goliath we see the aim and intent of the devil to accuse until confusion rids its opponent of spiritual sense. Goliath begins by saying, "Why have you come out to line up for battle?" Think of this ridiculous insinuation. The reason they came to line up for battle is to rid their land of the Philistines. To conquer them until they either surrender or are driven out.

The children of God with God's direction always conquer and accomplish their mission. This is like the devil trying to tell you not to get up, don't go to church, why fellowship with believers, and in the midst of your circumstances why would you show up to defend yourself? Do you have an answer? What would you say? Would these questions cause you to second-guess if they were coming from a frightful situation?

Remember, the devil is not a roaring lion, but he will act like one. He wants your full attention.

Next, Goliath says, "Am I not a Philistine and you the servants of Saul?" I am amazed as I see the Israelites listening to Goliath as though they had a previous agreement, that Goliath was going to be the moderator of the fight. Why listen to Goliath? Why not send six of your best horseman and archers to fill Goliath with arrows, and then give the terms of the fight? It would be something like, "We are the Children of the Most High God. God is on our side to deliver us from you uncircumcised Philistines. Surrender or we will destroy you." That sounds more like it!

So how about you? Have you been listening to the voices of discouragement? Who is moderating your battle? Look at what Goliath says to the Israelites, "Am I not a Philistine and you the servants of Saul? What's wrong with this statement? Who are the Israelites? Servants of a man or the children of God?

Focus on your position in Christ not your humanity. As long as the devil can get you to consider your humanity you will fight in your own strength. You can be certain that the devil will not remind you of your right standing with God. He will not encourage you to believe that you are indestructible, for then no weapon of his will prosper. The devil will cause you to roam or stray from the truth. The realm of reason is the territory of the devil.

You can resist the devil. Someone "special" other than yourself isn't needed. Next Goliath says, "Choose a man for yourselves; let him come down to me." You might say, "Why is this so wrong?" The truth is that any one under covenant can defeat the devil. It's just like Satan to challenge your stability by making you consider that only someone special can do the work. Every believer is empowered through Christ to enforce the victory of the Lord.

The devil will try to indoctrinate us to believe that only certain believers are specially equipped to handle his attacks. The moment he succeeds to divert your attention from who you are and what you are capable of doing, you lose by sheer default.

Move forward with certainty and confidence. Notice now that the devil uses the word "if" to finish off the psyche of the army of the Lord. "If he is able to fight with me and defeat me, then we will be your servants. If I am able to defeat him, then you will be our servants and serve us." These questions reveal uncertainty, the finishing touch that destroys confidence in God.

If God told Joshua that "no man is able to stand against you all the days of your life," then there is no question to discuss. Of course the Philistines will fail. There is no contest when God is fighting for you. However, through these accusations Satan has successfully diverted the armies of God from victory.

Invoke God's covenant promises to do the miraculous. At this point David enters as a delivery boy for his father. He comes at his father's request to see how the battle is going and to deliver food to his brothers and their captains. When David sees Goliath and hears his curses, his comment is simply, who is this uncircumcised Philistine that he should defy the armies of the Living God?

This is the first time covenant was mentioned in forty days. The truth about the servants of Saul is that they were in fact the armies of the living God. Even though they served Saul, they were God's army. How important it is for the devil to keep us from knowing who we are. The success of the enemy hangs in the balance of whether or not he can keep us ignorant or at least distracted. Isn't it interesting that if Goliath was so powerful, why didn't the Philistines overtake the Israelites when they wanted to? The obvious reason is that the devil is not all he makes himself out to be.

When I see David's question concerning Goliath, I am amazed at how unaffected he is at the accusations of Goliath. 1 Samuel 17:22-27 reads:

> *And David left his supplies in the hand of the supply keeper, ran to the army, and came and greeted his brothers. Then as he talked with them, there was the champion, the Philistine of Gath, Goliath by name, coming up from the armies of the Philistines; and he spoke according to the same words. So David heard them. And all the men of Israel, when they saw the man, fled from him and were dreadfully afraid. So the men*

> *of Israel said, "Have you seen this man who has come up? Surely he has come up to defy Israel; and it shall be that the man who kills him the king will enrich with great riches, will give him his daughter, and give his father's house exemption from taxes in Israel."*
>
> *Then David spoke to the men who stood by him, saying, "What shall be done for the man who kills this Philistine and takes away the reproach from Israel? For who is this uncircumcised Philistine, that he should defy the armies of the living God?"*
>
> *And the people answered him in this manner, saying," So shall it be done for the man who kills him."*

David hears the same words that the other men of the army have heard day and night for forty days. David views how the army reacts to the words of Goliath and hears the soldiers talking about the reward that the king of Israel offers for the man who defeats Goliath. David is more interested in the reward than giving a response first to what he thinks of Goliath.

I think that David's question to the men who have revealed the reward of the King is a question of amazement and excitement at the same time. It's **amazement** because it's hard for him to understand why a reward should be given for something that is so simple. It's **excitement** because the reward is very appealing for a single man who has been out in the desert watching sheep.

David is giving the men of the army of Israel the same kind of response that the apostles Peter and Paul would give us today if they saw how we handle our battles. He is shocked that no one has defeated the uncircumcised Philistine yet, and pleasantly surprised that with such a great reward no one has cashed in on it. How would Peter and Paul look at us today shying away from opportunities to witness, not knowing what to do concerning sicknesses that don't seem to leave and talking as if there isn't enough of God present to do the job? Wouldn't they walk into our churches and clean house?

They would challenge our doctrine, immediately loose people who have been bound and rebuke our lazy attitudes and unwillingness to get busy for God.

Would it not be fitting that religious people rise up against them reviling them for their pride and arrogance of heart? Can you see that many in our day would become furious if men like Peter or Paul brought correction to the body of Christ? And to think that David wasn't even bringing correction as much as he was surprised that no one had taken Goliath's challenge. Let's look at the accusations of David's brother:

> *Now Eliab his oldest brother heard when he spoke to the men; and Eliab's anger was aroused against David, and he said, "Why did you come down here? And with whom*

> have you left those few sheep in the wilderness? I know your pride and the insolence of your heart, for you have come down to see the battle."
> And David said, "What have I done now? Is there not a cause?" Then he turned from him toward another and said the same thing; and these people answered him as the first ones did.
> Now when the words which David spoke were heard, they reported them to Saul; and he sent for him. Then David said to Saul," Let no man's heart fail because of him; your servant will go and fight with this Philistine."
> (1 Sam. 17:28-32)

Don't look at a situation from the devil's perspective. Once the devil has successfully turned your attention from God toward the problem, it will be difficult to remain faithful to the truth. Eliab yields to pride and begins to hurl accusations at his own family. We cannot afford to see things through the devil's eyes or it will corrupt our whole view of life.

I like David's response, "What have I done now?" David's innocence is a byproduct of trust in God. David actually sees what the real problem is: *the men of the army of the Lord have missed the whole point of why they serve the Lord.*

David follows up by saying, "Is there not a cause?" In other words, isn't there a reason why someone should defend the righteousness of God. Covenant as we viewed in chapter four reveals the strength of partnership. If someone comes against you to fight, then they are coming against me. I will fight for and with you, and you will fight for and with me. God's honor is at stake. David cannot understand why someone will not defend the honor of God.

Do you see the similarities of our day? How long can we sit by and watch so much disaster in our world, especially when we have the solution for all of life's problems. Will no one accept the responsibility of standing in the gap for the gospel of Jesus Christ? If we don't do something to release God and reveal Him in the earth, who will?

In verse 32 David spoke to Saul that he would fight the Philistine. In this last day you will see many people who are not on the who's who list raised up to fight an effective battle. Saul commented in 1 Samuel 17:33-37:

> And Saul said to David,"You are not able to go against this Philistine to fight with him; for you are a youth, and he a man of war from his youth."
>
> But David said to Saul, "Your servant used to keep his father's sheep, and when a lion or a bear came and took a lamb out of the flock, I went out after it and struck it, and delivered the lamb from its mouth; and when it arose against me, I caught it by its beard, and struck and killed it. Your servant has killed both lion and bear; and this

uncircumcised Philistine will be like one of them, seeing he has defied the armies of the living God."

Moreover David said, "The LORD, who delivered me from the paw of the lion and from the paw of the bear, He will deliver me from the hand of this Philistine."

And Saul said to David, "Go, and the LORD be with you!"

Develop your faith. Practice living in the miraculous. Be prepared for the next crisis. As you can see, David used his personal experiences as a witness for the approval of the King. I cannot express enough how important it is to develop your faith in every area of your life. Don't wait until the crisis of life comes upon you to exercise your faith.

David had already proven his trust and reliability in the covenant of God. I personally think that David started at the top with the bear and the lion. By the time he tackled Goliath he was very comfortable in trusting God. It would be easy to say that the Lord delivered me from the paw of the lion and the paw of the bear if David had nothing to do with it, just like it's easy to be healed when your body doesn't hurt.

David was the one who went after the bear with his staff. He acted in faith by grabbing the beard of the lion. God was mighty for David when David exercised his faith. David knew that if he defended God, God would defend him.

The last part of this story that I want to relate to this chapter is the dialogue between David and Goliath. I'm always interested in watching the spirit of faith in people who trust in God. 1 Samuel 17:42-51 reads,

> *And when the Philistine looked about and saw David, he disdained him; for he was only a youth, ruddy and good-looking. So the Philistine said to David, "Am I a dog, that you come to me with sticks?" And the Philistine cursed David by his gods. And the Philistine said to David, "Come to me, and I will give your flesh to the birds of the air and the beasts of the field!"*
>
> *Then David said to the Philistine, "You come to me with a sword, with a spear, and with a javelin. But I come to you in the name of the LORD of hosts, the God of the armies of Israel, whom you have defied. This day the LORD will deliver you into my hand, and I will strike you and take your head from you. And this day I will give the carcasses of the camp of the Philistines to the birds of the air and the wild beasts of the earth, that all the earth may know that there is a God in Israel. Then all this assembly shall know that the LORD does not save with sword and spear; for the battle is the LORD's, and He will give you into our hands."*

> *So it was, when the Philistine arose and came and drew near to meet David, that David hurried and ran toward the army to meet the Philistine. Then David put his hand in his bag and took out a stone; and he slung it and struck the Philistine in his forehead, so that the stone sank into his forehead, and he fell on his face to the earth. So David prevailed over the Philistine with a sling and a stone, and struck the Philistine and killed him. But there was no sword in the hand of David. Therefore David ran and stood over the Philistine, took his sword and drew it out of its sheath and killed him, and cut off his head with it.*

The battle belongs to the Lord. Goliath, full of curses and insults, disdained David when he saw him. However, nothing the giant could do or say would move David away from his trust in God. After the giant revealed his intent to kill David, David spoke up with absolute confidence. He reveals why Goliath is in real trouble. Goliath only has a sword and shield. The Israelites will fight with the ability of God. David tells Goliath that he has defied the Lord. He obviously doesn't know what he is in for.

The fight is not against flesh and blood; it is the battle of God. What David says next is the battle cry of my heart. He is going to explain the position of the body of Christ in the earth. This is the reason why we have responsibility before God. David says, the

Lord will not only avenge Himself against Goliath, but also the entire camp of the Philistines. This will be done for two reasons. First, so that all the earth may know that there is a God in Israel. Second, that all the assembly shall know that the Lord does not save with sword and spear; for the battle is the Lord's.

The body of Christ is at a turning point just as the world is at a turning point in time. We must make an impact if the gospel message is to be heard throughout the world. The confrontation we see exhibited in the story of David and Goliath is to be natural for every believer within his or her sphere of influence.

In most cases it won't be as dramatic as displayed, however, it should be as effective. There will need to be leaders who will rise up to magnify God in the way presented in this story. A multitude of believers will have to see demonstrations of God's power to be convinced that the battle is the Lord's. The world deserves to see God as He really is.

Don't you love the attitude of David? He is not arrogant; there is such innocence to his confident demeanor. He is acting out of his relationship with God. He is not trying to prove anything for himself, yet he is standing up for what is right and just. He is 100% sure that God will fight for him if he presents himself before his enemy as a partner to righteousness. As wonderful as his presentation is, there is more to the victory. 1 Samuel 17:48-51 reads,

> *So it was, when the Philistine arose and came and drew near to meet David, that*

> *David hurried and ran toward the army to meet the Philistine.*
>
> *Then David put his hand in his bag and took out a stone; and he slung it and struck the Philistine in his forehead, so that the stone sank into his forehead, and he fell on his face to the earth.*
>
> *So David prevailed over the Philistine with a sling and a stone, and struck the Philistine and killed him. But there was no sword in the hand of David. Therefore David ran and stood over the Philistine, took his sword and drew it out of its sheath and killed him, and cut off his head with it.*

After David masterfully rebutted the words of Goliath, Goliath began to approach David. Everything up to this point is for naught if David chooses to back down to Goliath. Many Christians get to this place, but lose the fight for lack of initiative. Words and actions must be in harmony to merit the assistance of the Lord.

Are You Willing to Act on Your Faith?

You may be able to talk like you know what you're doing. However, when it's time for action, are you willing to exercise your faith? I believe with the story of David and Goliath that David never thought twice about whether or not he should follow through on his words. David knew he would win in the worst-case scenario. From the beginning, when David accepted the challenge, he fully expected to fight Goliath.

Would we have hoped that something would change the circumstances of the fight? Would we have looked for a way out? What kind of preparation caused David to be so strong and courageous?

Reiterating our scripture for this chapter, Jesus said, "If you abide in me and my words abide in you, you will ask what you desire and it will be done for you" (John 15: 7). There are two things that stand out to me when considering the life of David. First, his love for the word, and second, the time spent in fellowship with God.

There are two Psalms that typify the life of David. Notice the love David had for the Word of God in Psalm 119. I have selected certain verses for you to meditate on and see how important David believed God's Word to be:

- *v. 2: Blessed are those who keep His testimonies, who seek Him with the whole heart!*
- *v. 10: With my whole heart I have sought You; Oh, let me not wander from Your commandments!*
- *v. 15: I will meditate on your precepts, and contemplate Your ways.*
- *V. 16: I will delight myself in your statutes; I will not forget Your word.*

- v. 18: Open my eyes, that I may see wondrous things from Your law.
- v. 24: Your testimonies also are my delight and my counselors.
- v. 27: Make me understand the way of your precepts; so shall I meditate on your wonderful works.
- v. 37: Turn away my eyes from looking at worthless things, and revive me in your way.
- v. 47: And I will delight myself in your commandments, which I love. 48 My hands also I will lift up to your commandments, which I love, and I will meditate on your statutes.
- v. 50: This is my comfort in my affliction; For Your word has given me life.
- v. 59: I thought about my ways, and turned my feet to your testimonies.
- v. 62: At midnight I will rise to give thanks to You, Because of Your righteous judgments.
- v. 72: The law of your mouth is better to me than thousands of coins of gold and silver.
- v. 80: Let my heart be blameless regarding your statutes, that I may not be ashamed.
- v. 88: Revive me according to your lovingkindness, So that I may keep the testimony of your mouth.
- v. 89: Forever, O LORD, Your word is settled in heaven.
- v. 90: Your faithfulness endures to all generations; you established the earth, and it abides.

- *v. 93: I will never forget your precepts, for by them you have given me life.*
- *v. 97: Oh, how I love your law! It is my meditation all the day.*
- *v. 102: I have not departed from your judgments, for you yourself have taught me.*
- *v. 103: How sweet are your words to my taste, Sweeter than honey to my mouth!*
- *v. 104 Through Your precepts I understand; therefore I hate every false way.*
- *v. 105: Your word is a lamp to my feet and a light to my path.*
- *v. 106: I have sworn and confirmed that I will keep your righteous judgments.*
- *v. 114: You are my hiding place and my shield; I hope in your word.*
- *v. 127: Therefore I love your commandments More than gold, yes, than fine gold!*
- *v. 128: Therefore all your precepts concerning all things consider to be right; I hate every false way.*
- *v. 130: The entrance of your words gives light; it gives understanding to the simple.*
- *v. 131: I opened my mouth and panted, for I longed for your commandments.*
- *v. 137: Righteous are You, O LORD, and upright are your judgments.*
- *v. 138: Your testimonies, which you have commanded, are righteous and very faithful.*
- *v. 139: My zeal has consumed me, because my enemies have forgotten your words.*

- v. 140: *Your word is very pure; Therefore Your servant loves it.*
- v. 148: *My eyes are awake through the night watches that I may meditate on your word.*
- v. 159: *Consider how I love your precepts; revive me, O LORD, according to your loving kindness.*
- v. 160: *The entirety of your word is truth, and every one of your righteous judgments endures forever.*
- v. 161: *Princes persecute me without a cause, but my heart stands in awe of your word.*
- v. 162: *I rejoice at your word as one who finds great treasure.*
- v. 171: *My lips shall utter praise, for you teach me your statutes.*

David had a tremendous love for the Word of God. His respect and commitment to the word is what made him so powerful in the midst of confrontation. David never lost his point of reference. Because the word never departed from his eyes and mind, he was ever conscious of the heart or truth of the matter. Why be deceived by Goliath when it is so real to him that as an uncircumcised Philistine he is sure to fail. Not just remembering covenant, but living in it will make you immoveable.

We also need to discuss David's love for the presence of the Lord. I can imagine the longing for fellowship with someone intelligent, especially after spending so much time with the sheep.

The Lord is my light and my salvation; he protects me from danger-whom shall I fear? When evil men come to destroy me, they will stumble and fall! Yes, though a mighty army marches against me, my heart shall know no fear! I am confident that God will save me.

The one thing I want from God, the thing I seek most of all, is the privilege of meditating in his Temple, living in his presence every day of my life, delighting in his incomparable perfections and glory. There I'll be when troubles come. He will hide me. He will set me on a high rock out of reach of all my enemies. Then I will bring him sacrifices and sing his praises with much joy.

Listen to my pleading, Lord! Be merciful and send the help I need.

My heart has heard you say, "Come and talk with me, O my people." And my heart responds, "Lord, I am coming."

Oh, do not hide yourself when I am trying to find you. Do not angrily reject your servant. You have been my help in all my trials before; don't leave me now. Don't forsake me, O God of my salvation. For if my father and mother should abandon me, you would welcome and comfort me.

Tell me what to do, O Lord, and make it plain because I am surrounded by waiting enemies. Don't let them get me, Lord! Don't let me fall into their hands! For they accuse me

> *of things I never did, and all the while are plotting cruelty. I am expecting the Lord to rescue me again, so that once again I will see his goodness to me here in the land of the living.*
>
> *Don't be impatient. Wait for the Lord, and he will come and save you! Be brave, stouthearted, and courageous. Yes, wait and he will help you.* (Ps. 27 TLB)

Jesus said in John 15:7 that if we abide in Him and His word abides in us, we will ask what we will and it will be given to us. Abiding in His word is the time we take to meditate truth. Abiding in Him is fellowshipping with the Lord. Time is necessary to develop any relationship. How important it becomes, when the pressures begin to surround us, that we really know the Lord.

Spend time abiding in Him. It's one thing to know about Him, but entirely another thing to *know* Him. The benefits of knowing what God has said and then knowing that He will back it up is crucial to your relationship. If someone says they have faith without fellowship, you watch, they will struggle when the pressure's on.

The reason why everything God says is so comforting to me is because from my time with Him, I'm confident that He would never leave me alone. Everything that promotes knowing about God through knowledge is time spent in the word. Although my studies are first and foremost, and learning about God through the experiences of those written in the Bible is faith building, there still is nothing like spending time with God for yourself.

Whether praying in your known language or praying in other tongues, singing in the spirit in psalms and hymns and spiritual songs or just being quiet while you wait on Him; learning to trust Him can only be obtained by spending time between you and God.

I am truly grateful to the Holy Spirit for teaching me some things that are producing fruit. The Holy Spirit has led each step that I have taken as a soul progression in the things of God. Revelation has been continual as I pray in the Holy Ghost. John said in 1 John 2:27, "But the anointing which you have received from Him abides in you, and you do not need that anyone teach you; but as the same anointing teaches you concerning all things, and is true, and is not a lie, and just as it has taught you, you will abide in Him."

The presence of God was the very reality of God that man was separated from because of the wall of sin. Man without God gropes around without purpose and direction. We do, however, have a wonderful end of the story in Christ. Even though the first man, Adam, lost the blessed privilege of communion with God, the last Adam completely restored what was lost. Jesus paved a way into the Holy of Holies. With His precious blood, which is ever pres-ent at the mercy seat, access has been provided into the very presence of God our Father.

We are not alone, forsaken or lost. Never again do we need to feel forsaken and lost. The abiding presence like an overcoat, or as an unseen companion will forever host us through this valley of the shadow of death to a greater understanding and experience of God. If David, so full of confidence from his time spent with God and in complete understanding of covenant rights and privileges, could so easily defeat Goliath, then it's time to ask ourselves:

- What would it be like for sons of God to assume their duty as God's representatives in the earth?
- Will the church ever be so confident of God's ability and faithfulness to accomplish everything that we presently long for?
- What are the possibilities of believing God?

Living in the Miraculous

- Stop listening to the devil's perspective.

- Stop being distracted by the devil's appeal to natural reason.

- Start believing that the battle belongs to the Lord.

- Start acting on your faith.

- Start abiding in Christ daily by spending time with Him in worship, the Word, prayer, praying in the Spirit, and practicing the presence of God in every relationship and circumstance.

Conclusion

THE MIRACULOUS—GUARANTEED!

Consider now how short the time is for us to live in the miraculous. Jesus said: *"Take heed that no one deceives you. For many will come in My name, saying, 'I am the Christ,' and will deceive many. And you will hear of wars and rumors of wars. See that you are not troubled; for all these things must come to pass, but the end is not yet. For nation will rise against nation, and kingdom against kingdom. And there will be famines, pestilences, and earthquakes in various places. All these are the beginning of sorrows.*

"Then they will deliver you up to tribulation and kill you, and you will be hated by all nations for My name's sake. And then

> many will be offended, will betray one another, and will hate one another. Then many false prophets will rise up and deceive many. And because lawlessness will abound, the love of many will grow cold. But he who endures to the end shall be saved. And this gospel of the kingdom will be preached in all the world as a witness to all the nations, and then the end will come. (Matt. 24:4-14)

The apostle Paul wrote:

> But mark this: There will be terrible times in the last days. People will be lovers of themselves, lovers of money, boastful, proud, abusive, disobedient to their parents, ungrateful, unholy, without love, unforgiving, slanderous, without self-control, brutal, not lovers of the good, treacherous, rash, conceited, lovers of pleasure rather than lovers of God- having a form of godliness but denying its power. Have nothing to do with them. (2 Tim. 3:1-5 NIV)

Time as we know it is definitely drawing to a close. Even with recent events, our nation is encountering difficulties that have never been presented on this scale before. If history repeats itself, then during hard and difficult times the world cries out for a savior.

What brand of Christianity do you think will meet the need of the world?

To what degree will the supernatural play a part in this last hour of the church?

The answer is simple.

As children of the living God, we must live in the miraculous. We cannot fail unless we choose to live by the visible instead of the invisible...unless we choose not to act in faith.

When we act in faith on the irrefutable, covenant promises of God's Word, we live in the miraculous, and we proclaim that Jesus is Lord and Savior until He comes!

ABOUT THE AUTHOR

Jim Hockaday was born again at four years of age. Experiencing the call of God at this time and the desire to preach, Jim led many to the Lord during his childhood. After graduation from Wheaton College in 1983, he traveled with several Christian music groups, including the Spurlows, Truth, and the Living Word Singers.

When God put in Jim's heart a strong desire to know more of Him, he attended Rhema Bible Training Center and graduated in 1988. Immediately following graduation, he joined the Rhema Singers and Band and traveled extensively with Rev. Kenneth E. Hagin and the group for nearly seven years; during the last several years he had the management responsibility of the Group. Jim was the Coordinator of Prayer and Healing School for Kenneth Hagin Ministries, completing his tenth year in May 2004.

He founded *Jim Hockaday Ministries, Inc.* in 1991, and now travels and ministers full time in churches at home and abroad.

Jim is the author of several books, one of which is the best selling book, **Until I Come...** and the most recent release, **Where Does God Fit In?**

Jim, his wife Erin (a 1991 graduate of Rhema Bible Training Center and member of the Rhema Singers and Band for two and a half years), reside in the Denver area.

Books By Jim Hockaday

Until I Come
The works I do you shall do also!

Living In the Miraculous
This is the time to live in the miraculous! Let's do it!

Where Does God Fit In?
Anywhere you let Him! Stop wondering and start reading!

The Miraculous Gospel of John with Commentary
Let your life resemble...the love and power of Jesus!

Miracles NOW!
Nuggets to Inspire your faith!

Identity Crisis
Let God settle the age-old question...what is man?

For more information on books and resources by Jim Hockaday, visit his website at: www.jimhockaday.com.

CONTACT INFORMATION

To contact the Author please write:

Jim Hockaday Ministries, Inc.
P.O. Box 729
Castle Rock, CO 80104

You can also visit us on the web at
www.jimhockaday.com

We welcome your comments, prayer requests, and especially your miracles!